CW00816444

THE

ILLUMINATED

BREATH

Transform Your Physical, Cognitive & Emotional Well-Being by Harnessing the Science of Ancient Yoga Breath Practices

DYLAN WERNER

VICTORY BELT PUBLISHING

Las Vegas

First published in 2021 by Victory Belt Publishing Inc.

ISBN-13: 978-1-628604-23-8

The author is not a licensed practitioner, physician, or medical professional and offers no medical diagnoses, treatments, suggestions, or counseling. The information presented herein has not been evaluated by the U.S. Food and Drug Administration, and it is not intended to diagnose, treat, cure, or prevent any disease. Full medical clearance from a licensed physician should be obtained before beginning or modifying any diet, exercise, or lifestyle program, and physicians should be informed of all nutritional changes.

The author/owner claims no responsibility to any person or entity for any liability, loss, or damage caused or alleged to be caused directly or indirectly as a result of the use, application, or interpretation of the information presented herein.

Cover design and illustrations by Dylan Werner

Interior design by Kat Lannom

Printed in Canada

TC 0121

CONTENTS

claims, the information was incorrect, misleading, or contrived. Still more often, only a brief description would be given for the practice with a generalized reference to a few physical benefits.

Thankfully, along this journey, I found a few teachers who demonstrated these breathing practices and explained the physiology and benefits supporting them. I am so grateful to the teachers who opened the doors of knowledge to me and pointed me in the right direction. One of the hardest challenges in the pursuit of knowledge is knowing which questions to ask. Sometimes finding the right answers to the wrong questions can leave us even more lost than we were when and where we began.

As I dove deeper into the breath practice, I began to open myself more to the emotional and energetic effects of breathing. Initially, I was closed to anything that resembled spirituality. Many of the yogic philosophies didn't appeal to me because I didn't understand how they were useful. Early on, I found the concept of *chakras* (subtle body energy centers) beautiful but didn't know how the knowledge of them could help me. I owe gratitude to my teachers for holding my hand and showing me what I was incapable of seeing on my own. But even as I broadened my understanding of *prana* (the Sanskrit word relating to energy) and the physiological effects of the breath, it took me years to grasp their correlations. Even now, as I say I understand that these are two sides of the same coin, I know I am only an infant on this journey to truly comprehend the potential that the breath has to influence our lives in significant and transformative ways.

EASTERN PHILOSOPHY MEETS WESTERN SCIENCE

I began to recognize in my study of breathing that I was traveling down parallel paths. The first explored the physiological effects through modern science; the second sought out the energetic movements of *prana* through Eastern and yogic philosophies. I ultimately realized that these two systems were essentially talking about the same thing in different languages. What was even more fascinating to me was that the breath influenced the Eastern and Western systems in the same way.

The autonomic nervous system can be viewed as our Western system of energy. It influences our emotional reactions and physical responses to situations such as fear and danger or comfort and safety. It maintains internal stability and controls all our major organs and cardiorespiratory system. The autonomic nervous system regulates these functions with its two sub-branches. Most of you are probably familiar with the sympathetic and parasympathetic nervous systems, but you might not know that the autonomic nervous system can be broken down into three branches using the polyvagal theory. Through this theory, we gain a deeper understanding of the nervous system's relationship to emotions and social engagement. The autonomic nervous system functions to maintain homeostasis. Too much in one area creates a deficiency in another, which can cause dysfunctions and imbalances both physically and emotionally.

The breath has an immediate effect on the nervous system and a direct influence to balance it. Inhaling stimulates the sympathetic nervous system, and exhaling stimulates the parasympathetic nervous system. When we begin to understand that the autonomic nervous system directly controls our emotions, mood, heart rate, digestion, sex life, and so much more and that our breath can effect change in this system, we start to realize how much influence we have over our physical bodies and our emotions.

Yoga draws these maps slightly differently. The maps help us see the same landscape but through a different point of reference. Imagine viewing a map of California depicting the state's topography, another map that details the state's roadways, and a third that delineates city lines. All three maps give us a different insight into the state as we drive up the coast. It doesn't matter which map we are looking at; we are traveling in the same direction.

The same is true as we look at the different yogic energy systems. These yoga philosophies help us identify the imbalances in our lives and show us which way to move energetically to find balance, peace, and harmony. For example, we can use our knowledge of the *gunas,* which explain the physical manifestation of energy that exists in all things, to understand our imbalances. The three *gunas* represent the continuous flow of energetic movement, from ascending and expanding to descending and contracting. We see these currents of energy expressed in nature and in ourselves. The *gunas* represent our physical and emotional attributes and offer a different kind of map to help us understand the self for the purpose of living a more conscious and healthy life. The energy of the *gunas* flows with the breath in the same way that the autonomic nervous system does. When we inhale, our energy ascends and expands, and when we exhale, it descends and contracts.

As we navigate our environment, we learn how to use these maps, and when we feel lost, these systems might give us insight into which direction we should travel.

In addition to profoundly influencing over our emotions, the breath significantly affects our physiology. With only our breath, we can change the pH of our blood, speed up or slow down our heart rate, lower our blood pressure, increase our ability to focus and form new memories, boost our athletic performance, and more.

So the big question is, how can we use the breath, which is always readily available, no matter where we are or what we are doing, to manifest our intentions and move us toward our goals? Every breathing technique or *pranayama* practice has unique qualities and means to affect the mind and body. Typically, a single breathing technique conveys several effects and has an abundance of applications. When we understand what the breath does, how it does those things, and why, we can customize each breathing technique; combine several techniques, pulling out just the components of these exercises that physically or energetically bring us closer to our goal and intention; and sequence these breathing practices in a way that accentuates and amplifies their effects.

I have been developing this method of breath sequencing and sharing it with thousands of people all over the world for the past several years. It is not a traditional approach to *pranayama,* and it is much more intricate than most breathing practices you'll find. What I am offering here is both new and ancient. I don't try to separate the knowledge that has been passed down for thousands of years from the latest science and physiological discoveries. Instead, I use the approach that yoga has taught me through my years of practice and study: Everything is connected and interdependent. There is no separation between the mind, body, and spirit. The clear unifying factor is our breath. Only by taking a holistic approach will we find comprehensive results.

Although respiration seems simple—there is only an inhalation, an inner retention, an exhalation, and an outer retention—these four parts are so incredibly complex and intricate that changing one element even slightly can impact almost every aspect of life, just like each color in the rainbow comes from some combination of red, yellow, and blue. When we discover the possibilities the breath has to offer, we become like artists learning for the first time that we can blend these colors together. For many of us, the breath is a tool we never knew how to use—or never even knew we had.

HOW TO USE THIS BOOK

This book is broken into five sections. The first section guides you through the physiology of the breath, the anatomical structures involved in breathing, and the physical effects that the breath has on the body and mind. For non–anatomy nerds, this information can be challenging to absorb. I have made sure to highlight key physiological concepts throughout the book so that the next time you see something science related, it is explained again, possibly in a new way that you may relate to better. The physiological effects and explanations are interwoven into every breathing practice so that by the time you finish this book, you will be well versed in these concepts.

The second section discusses what I view as the "systems of balance" and how energy travels through the body through the influence of our breath. We begin with the nervous system, both how it functions physically throughout the body and how it affects us emotionally, moving through different theories that can help us understand our reactions and tendencies in situations that arise from our inner and outer environments. Then we explore the Eastern viewpoint using yoga philosophies and how yoga outlines the way energy moves.

The third section on *pranayama* and the concepts that are associated with the yogic breath practice continues with the Eastern philosophy. Each *pranayama* practice is explained and broken down to illustrate the technique, its energetic and emotional effects, its physiological effects, and its applications.

These first three sections establish a foundation for understanding the breath. The fourth section explores how to take these *pranayama* practices and breathing concepts, modify them to our intention, and sequence them to accomplish the purpose of our practice.

The final section outlines ten breath sequences that I created, covering several aspects and conditions of life where the breath can be utilized as a powerful tool to manifest positive change and influence health and well-being. Throughout these sequences, I offer insights I've gathered from my eclectic life and share some wisdom that we all already know but probably need to hear again.

I want to clarify that this book is not just for yoga practitioners. It is intended for anyone who desires to live a better, happier, and healthier life. I use several yoga concepts, Sanskrit terms, ancient wisdom, and *pranayama* techniques to bring us deeper into aspects of yoga that have been practiced for thousands of years. I do not try to push any of the metaphysical ideas of energy, or *prana,* or claim the physical existence of these yogic concepts. I also don't suggest that they do not exist. I illustrate each of them in a way that we can use to understand the underlying emotional conditions of our lives and how our energetic tendencies can be drawn toward one extreme or another. These yoga philosophies give us another lens through which to view parts of our lives that we may be unaware of but can be deep-seated sources of pain and suffering. A map is only useful if we know how to use it and if it relates to where we want to go. I believe these maps provide valuable information on how to restore balance to our lives.

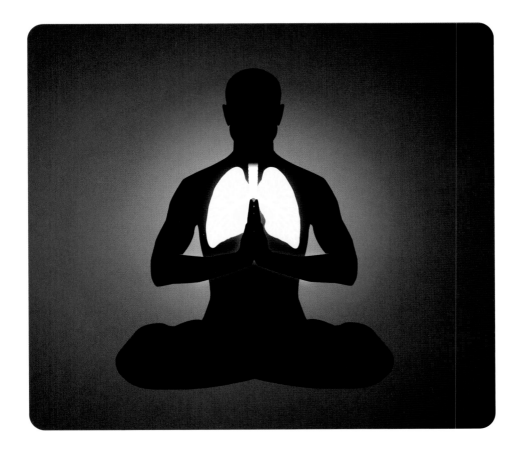

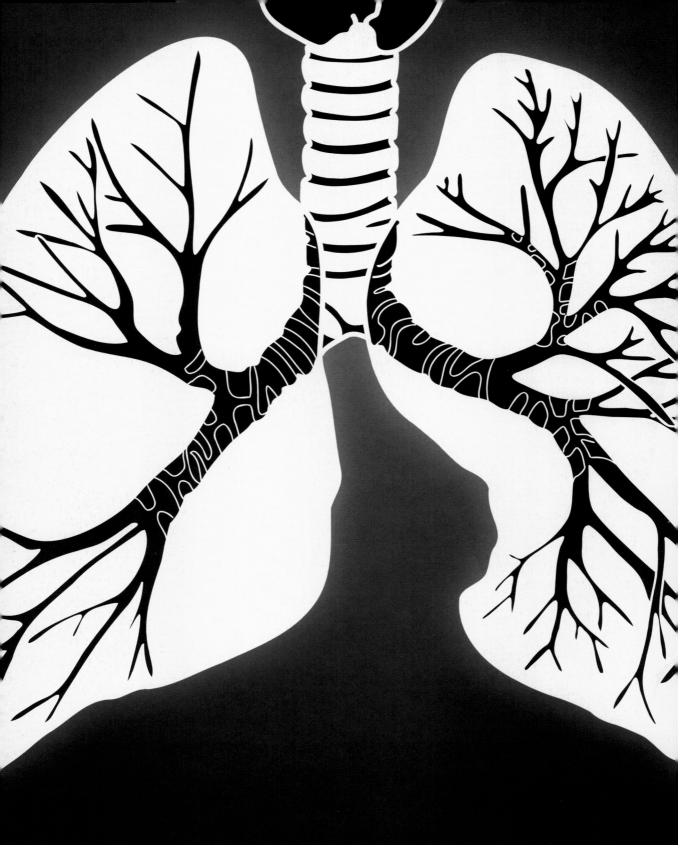

[SECTION 1]
THE PHYSIOLOGY OF BREATHING

Why do we breathe? It might sound like a silly question. We breathe to live, of course. We all know that, of all the things we can't survive without, our breath is the thing we need the most. Breathing delivers oxygen to our cells so that they can function, create energy, and remove waste. But breathing has so many more responsibilities than just exchanging gases. The breath affects everything from our cardiovascular system to the balance and function of our nervous system. It affects how we deal with difficult situations. Breathing helps maintain and regulate blood pH and affects how we fight off illness and disease. Good breathing practices can significantly contribute to improved athletic performance and recovery and can even help with memory, learning, and concentration. We can use the breath to boost our sex drive, digestion, and so much more!

As a yoga teacher and educator, I instruct my students to avoid cues like "breathe" and, even worse, "just breathe." If we are always breathing and we'll die if we stop, chances are that even the ones holding their breath will eventually take a breath, whether their instructors tell them to or not. It's not "just breathing" that's important; it's *how* we breathe. If our breath has the ability to affect nearly every facet of our mental and physical well-being, then how we breathe is how we gain control of and influence our well-being.

CELLULAR RESPIRATION

We breathe primarily for the purpose of taking in oxygen through inhalation and eliminating waste gases through exhalation. Both sides of the breath cycle support cellular respiration—the process cells undergo to create energy. The complicated chemistry behind this process can be difficult to understand, but the basic idea is simple. The food we eat is broken down through digestion to make fuel for our cells. The primary fuel is glucose. Glucose and oxygen combine inside little organelles in the cells called mitochondria. The mitochondria then convert glucose and oxygen to carbon dioxide, water, and energy. The energy comes in the form of adenosine triphosphate, or ATP, which the body is able to use for fuel. And this gives the lungs their main job, which is to bring in oxygen to facilitate cellular respiration and breathe out carbon dioxide and water. Typically, we don't think we are expelling water, but if you exhale into your hand, you can feel the humidity. A more tangible illustration of this phenomenon involves fogging up a cold piece of glass by breathing on it. The fog is nothing more than the water and heat from your breath.

CELLULAR RESPIRATION

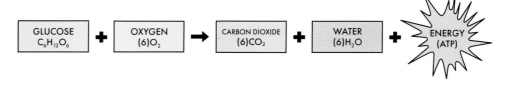

| GLUCOSE $C_6H_{12}O_6$ | + | OXYGEN $(6)O_2$ | → | CARBON DIOXIDE $(6)CO_2$ | + | WATER $(6)H_2O$ | + | ENERGY (ATP) |

Cellular respiration combines glucose and oxygen to create energy. Carbon dioxide and water are produced as by-products of the chemical reaction.

Breathing also plays a considerable role in regulating the pH levels of our blood. Normal blood pH is 7.4, but it varies from 7.35 to 7.45. As we breathe faster, our pH levels rise, and we become more alkaline. As we slow the breath down, our pH levels drop, and we become more acidic. Our bodies continuously monitor and regulate our blood pH by varying the rate and depth of our breathing as needed. If we're at rest, our breath is slow and shallow, but if we go for a run, we breathe faster and deeper. That more rapid breathing reflects the body's increase in both energy use and production of carbon dioxide, which lowers blood pH (making it more acidic). So, to regulate that, we need to exhale all that extra carbon dioxide.

THE PH SCALE

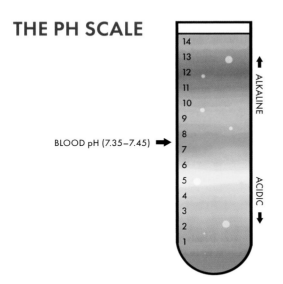

BLOOD pH (7.35–7.45)

ALKALINE

ACIDIC

pH stands for the potential of hydrogen. The scale ranges from 0 to 14, with 0 being highly acidic, such as battery acid; 14 being highly alkaline, such as liquid drain cleaner; and 7 being neutral, such as water. Our blood maintains a sensitive pH balance between 7.35 and 7.45. If the blood becomes too acidic or alkaline, it can result in serious health problems. Death occurs if blood pH drops below 6.8 or rises above 7.8.

THE CARBONIC-BICARBONATE BUFFER SYSTEM

Through its normal metabolic process, the body releases hydrogen ions (H+), which make the blood more acidic. If there are too many hydrogen ions in the blood, the body combines them with bicarbonate (HCO_3−) to form carbonic acid (H_2CO_3). It is able to break down the carbonic acid into carbon dioxide (CO_2) and water (H_2O), which are then exhaled, resulting in a rise in alkalinity. But if we become too alkaline, carbon dioxide combines with water in the blood to make carbonic acid, and the blood becomes more acidic to neutralize the excessive alkalinity.[1] To keep it simple going forward, I will simply reference the effect that carbon dioxide has on the body and call it carbon dioxide.

BUFFER SYSTEM

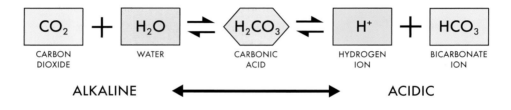

The carbonic-bicarbonate buffer system maintains the pH level of the blood. If the blood is too acidic, with too many free hydrogen ions, then the hydrogen ions combine with bicarbonate to create carbonic acid, which is then broken down into water and carbon dioxide to be expelled via the lungs. If the blood is too alkaline, water and carbon dioxide combine to create carbonic acid, and the process is reversed.

Breathing is controlled by our autonomic nervous system and our central nervous system, meaning that it is generally an involuntary process that we can override to a certain extent. (Turn to Section 2 for more on the nervous system.) Therefore, we can voluntarily hyperventilate and raise our blood pH levels until we feel dizzy and light-headed, have tingling sensations in the face and body, and have muscle spasms in the hands and feet. If we are breathing hard and fast for a long time, we might eventually pass out. We can also try to hold our breath for a long time until our diaphragm starts to spasm and we experience an intense sensation known as air hunger. If we are trained and disciplined, we might be able to fight the urge to breathe until we pass out. Usually, though, the autonomic nervous system takes control before we lose consciousness and restores our natural breathing. In most cases, we don't want to bring ourselves to such extremes willingly, but our ability to consciously change the rate, rhythm, and depth of the breath gives us the power to use the breath as an effective tool for bettering our health, emotional state, and well-being.

I like to do a little experiment with my students when I teach them about breathing, and the results are generally the same in every group. I have them breathe very fast and deep, usually through the mouth, for about a minute. After a minute, when they are feeling light-headed and dizzy, I ask them if they are feeling that way because they have too much oxygen to the brain. The majority answer yes.

We think we need to breathe more to get more oxygen into our cells, but it is actually carbon dioxide that plays an essential role in making this exchange happen. Also, we can't get more oxygen into our cells just by taking in more air. The main reason is that our blood is already fully saturated with oxygen. Normal blood oxygen saturation for a healthy person is between 95 and 99 percent; this means that the hemoglobin on the red blood cells is already carrying as much oxygen as it can handle. Trying to squeeze in more oxygen doesn't result in any improvement, just as trying to squeeze one or two more passengers into a packed subway car wouldn't result in any improvement to the mode of transportation or the harmony of those being transported.

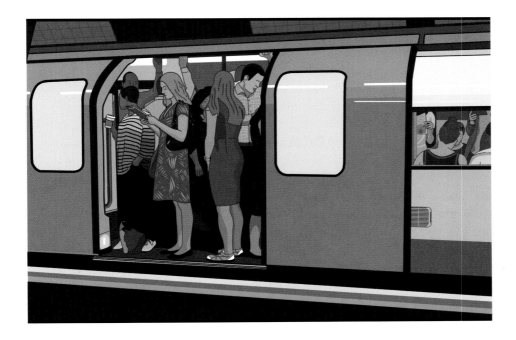

A common myth is that if we breathe more, we get more oxygen. Normal blood oxygen saturation for a healthy person is between 95 and 99 percent. The circulatory system acts like a series of subway lines, and our oxygen-carrying red blood cells are like subway cars, delivering oxygen to the body. If the cars are full, trying to cram in more people isn't going to help. Instead, we need to increase the number of cars (red blood cells) and the efficiency of getting people on and off the train.

CARBON DIOXIDE AND THE BOHR EFFECT

Why do we feel dizzy when we breathe too fast? To answer this question, we need to understand the role of carbon dioxide. First, carbon dioxide plays a significant role in every breath we take. It's a common misconception that we breathe because we are running low on oxygen. We are stimulated to breathe based on how much carbon dioxide is in our blood. (The exception is people who have chronic respiratory problems, such as emphysema or chronic obstructive pulmonary disease, or COPD, who live with abnormally high levels of carbon dioxide and breathe based on low oxygen.) As we hold our breath, chemoreceptors sense the decrease in pH (more acidic) and the increase in carbon dioxide; this stimulates us to take the next breath. The higher the carbon dioxide levels, the stronger the desire is to breathe. This urge is why it gets harder and harder to hold our breath for a long time. Generally, when we experience that strong urge to breathe, we still have plenty of oxygen in our blood. When I measure my blood oxygen levels while holding my breath, I don't see a drop in oxygen saturation until around three minutes of retention, and this is long after I have an urge to breathe. The time it takes for SpO_2 (peripheral capillary oxygen saturation) levels to drop varies from person to person and depends on a variety of factors, the main one being how many red blood cells are in the body.

As we breathe, the hemoglobin in the red blood cells binds to oxygen as it passes through the lungs, creating oxyhemoglobin. The red blood cells then go out to the body to supply our cells with oxygen. The only problem is that for the red blood cells to release oxygen, oxyhemoglobin needs carbon dioxide to increase blood acidity to facilitate the cellular exchange. This physiological event is called the Bohr effect, named after Nobel Prize–winning Danish physician Christian Bohr. The Bohr effect states, "Hemoglobin's oxygen binding affinity is inversely related both to acidity and to the concentration of carbon dioxide."[2] Hemoglobin is an iron-rich oxygen-carrying protein inside red blood cells. There are about 270 million hemoglobin molecules per red blood cell, and each hemoglobin molecule can carry four oxygen molecules. That means each red blood cell can hold over a billion oxygen molecules. As carbon dioxide levels rise due to cellular respiration, blood pH becomes more acidic, and the bond between the oxygen and hemoglobin is loosened so that oxygen can be released into the cells. If carbon dioxide levels are low and blood pH is high, the red blood cells can't release oxygen to the cells.

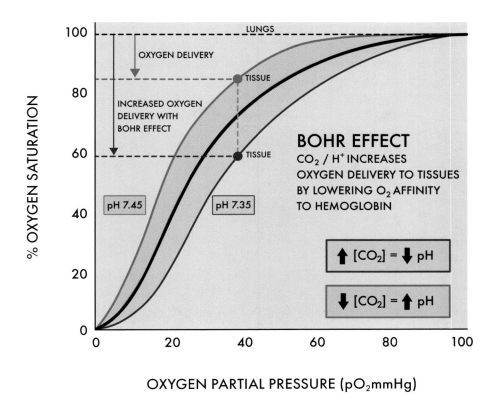

Oxygen has a strong affinity (attraction) to hemoglobin, the oxygen-carrying protein component of the red blood cells. This affinity allows oxygen to bind to hemoglobin in the lungs easily. When the oxygen gets to the tissues, it needs to be able to be released from the red blood cells. As carbon dioxide increases in the tissues and blood, blood pH decreases. The decrease in pH lowers oxygen's affinity to hemoglobin, and the oxygen is released to fuel the cells. The Bohr effect shows that higher carbon dioxide levels and a lower blood pH create better oxygenation of tissues.

The body is the ultimate "use it or lose it" system. Whatever we do, our bodies work to support us. If we run, our bodies will work in a way to help us become better at running. Our leg muscles will get stronger, our tendons will become more bouncy and elastic, and our endurance will increase. If we practice sitting on the couch, our bodies are going to get really good at sitting on the couch. The body's main concern is survival, and our survival is dependent on having the energy to fuel the body as well as store reserves to get more energy when fuel starts to run low. Muscles take a lot of energy, which is why our muscles atrophy when we stop exercising. Fat is the body's way to store energy, which is why it stores any excess it receives as adipose tissue.

Every second, approximately 2 to 2.5 million of our red blood cells die, and about the same number are created in our bone marrow to replace them. Those red blood cells will live for three to four months before they are replaced with new ones based on the body's current demands. "Current demands" are important to understand. Our bodies respond to what we've been doing; it doesn't know what we are *going to* need to do. If we are breathing too much (chronic over-breathing, which I'll explain a little later), our carbon dioxide levels stay low, and the red blood cells can't release oxygen. As a result, the body thinks it has too many red blood cells, so it doesn't replace them when they die. We are then left with the bare minimum number of red blood cells we need to survive. In this state, if we decided to go for a run, we would become winded rather quickly. Chronic over-breathers also can't hold their breath very long. When they do, their SpO_2 levels drop quickly because they don't have extra red blood cells circulating to meet the new demand.

So carbon dioxide stimulates us to breathe and allows oxygen to be released from the red blood cells so that it can be used by the muscles, organs, and every other cell in the body. Carbon dioxide also opens our airways, which is called bronchodilation, so we can breathe better. It expands our blood vessels, called vasodilation, which lowers blood pressure and allows the blood to perfuse our extremities with less effort by the heart. The opposite happens when carbon dioxide levels are low (a state known as hypocapnia). Our airways get smaller and our blood vessels constrict. As carbon dioxide levels decrease, the blood vessels going to the brain constrict. In turn, the brain receives significantly less blood and oxygen, which is why we feel light-headed and dizzy when we hyperventilate. This familiar response is not from too much oxygen; it's from too *little.* Bringing more oxygen into the brain makes us feel clear, aware, and focused.

Increasing carbon dioxide levels through breathing less offers many amazing benefits, which is why so many of the practices in this book are focused on holding the breath, slowing components of the breath, or simply creating good habits of breathing less. The majority of people who over-breathe are not aware that they do it. When you go out in public, notice how many people are breathing through their mouths. Anyone who is mouth breathing is over-breathing. The nose creates about 50 percent more airflow restriction than the mouth. In other words, if we are breathing through our mouths, we are breathing twice as much as we should, and it's a downward spiral from there. Mouth breathing leads to lower levels of carbon dioxide, which means the red blood cells can't release oxygen into our tissues, and our cells aren't adequately perfused. The red blood cells return to the lungs still carrying their full oxygen load. The body recognizes this as a waste of energy, and since making new red blood cells takes energy, it doesn't replace those returning cells because it doesn't think it needs to. This means less oxygen-carrying hemoglobin, which means anytime we do anything, we'll need to breathe faster and deeper, which again lowers carbon dioxide levels. And, unfortunately, this cycle continues.

THE UPPER RESPIRATORY SYSTEM

The mouth is made for talking, eating, and drinking, and the nose is designed for breathing. There are breathing exercises that involve inhaling through the mouth and exercises where we purposefully exhale as much carbon dioxide as possible. I will talk about why we do those exercises later. Otherwise, nasal breathing is the proper way to breathe.

Respiration starts with the nose. Generally, one nostril is restricted, while the other is mostly clear. About every four hours, the inside of one nostril becomes swollen, and the other opens up. This phenomenon is called the nasal cycle, and about 80 percent of people experience this switching of one nostril or the other being closed to some degree. The nasal cycle works to alternate the workload of breathing so that the mucous membranes inside the nose don't dry out, and it also helps improve our sense of smell by allowing air to enter both fast and slowly through the clear and partially restricted nostrils.

Beyond smelling and down-regulating air intake, the nose has many other functions. It is responsible for warming, humidifying, and filtering the air we breathe in, moving air along the respiratory mucosa inside the nasal cavity.[3] The lungs require warm moist air, regardless of how cold it might be outside or how high the air-conditioning is cranked. But one of the most amazing functions of the nose is its ability to increase levels of nitric oxide through inspiration, which is something we don't get from mouth breathing.

UPPER RESPIRATORY TRACT

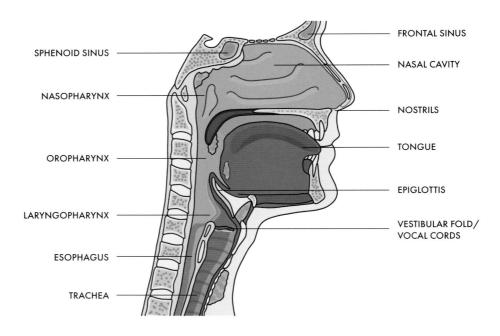

SPHENOID SINUS

NASOPHARYNX

OROPHARYNX

LARYNGOPHARYNX

ESOPHAGUS

TRACHEA

FRONTAL SINUS

NASAL CAVITY

NOSTRILS

TONGUE

EPIGLOTTIS

VESTIBULAR FOLD/ VOCAL CORDS

THE SIGNIFICANCE OF NITRIC OXIDE

Nitric oxide is a signaling molecule that is made in the lining of the blood vessels, in the nasal cavity, and in the paranasal sinus. As we inhale through the nose, nitric oxide is carried into our lungs and through the rest of the body. Nitric oxide has a long list of health benefits:

- It works alongside carbon dioxide to assist with oxygen binding and release and increases cellular oxygen uptake by 10 to 20 percent.

- It is a smooth muscle relaxer and vasodilator, working to regulate and lower blood pressure and improve circulation and control vascular tone.

- It increases the health and elasticity of blood vessels, lowers cholesterol, and decreases plaque buildup, which has a significant impact on cardiovascular health.

People with low levels of nitric oxide are more likely to have cardiac problems such as high blood pressure and heart attacks, as well as an increased risk of strokes. As we get older, nitric oxide production naturally decreases, so working to increase nitric oxide levels through proper breathing as well as diet is vital for our overall health.

PARANASAL SINUSES

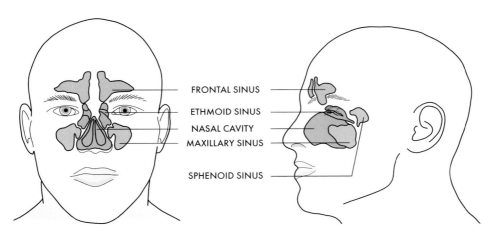

FRONTAL SINUS

ETHMOID SINUS

NASAL CAVITY

MAXILLARY SINUS

SPHENOID SINUS

Along with general cardiovascular health, nitric oxide is one of the miracle molecules for increasing strength and fitness and decreasing recovery time. Because it's a vasodilator, having higher levels of nitric oxide means that more blood and oxygen can perfuse our muscles; increased circulation also helps reduce lactic acid buildup, delayed-onset muscle soreness (DOMS), and fatigue. Nitric oxide promotes cell proliferation, which is the growth and reproduction of cells. It also helps increase oxygen delivery to the mitochondria, which gives us much more energy to be active. Nitric oxide works to decrease inflammation, increase the production of antioxidants, and improve immune system function.[4]

In addition to these physical benefits, nitric oxide is a powerful neuro-transmitter that aids in the rapid communication between brain cells, which increases learning capacity, concentration, and memory. Because nitric oxide isn't produced during mouth breathing, mouth breathers experience a massive decrease in levels of nitric oxide. Multiple studies have shown that children who mouth breathe are more likely to have learning disabilities than children who nasal breathe.[5] Ultimately, the importance of both nitric oxide and nasal breathing with regard to learning is incontrovertible.

When we breathe in slowly through the nose, we take in more nitric oxide than when we breathe fast. Slow nasal breathing has a profound calming and relaxing effect, with impacts on the brain that are similar to those of dopamine and serotonin, two other types of neurotransmitters. Nitric oxide also works to regulate the sympathetic nervous system, which governs our cardiovascular system and our fight-or-flight response, as you'll learn about later. Its ability to help control our reaction to perceived danger lessens the effect we feel when we are afraid, stressed, or nervous. This is why our bodies and minds are best served by taking slow, calm breaths when we find ourselves in stressful or scary situations.

Because nitric oxide both is a vasodilator and positively influences the autonomic nervous system, it helps increase libido and sexual function.[6] Sex drive and sexual function are highly emotionally based. Our autonomic nervous system has a significant impact on sexual function in both men and women. Stress is the leading cause of sexual and erectile dysfunction, because when we are stressed, the sympathetic nervous system overrides the parasympathetic nervous system. There needs to be sufficient parasympathetic tone for a man to have an erection and for a woman to produce vaginal lubrication. Nitric oxide helps calm the mind, alleviate stress, and reestablish healthy function of the parasympathetic nervous system. The other chief function of nitric oxide, vasodilation, acts to increase blood flow to the genitalia. Men get a harder erection, and women get more blood flow to the clitoris, creating more pressure, more sensitivity, and more intense orgasms. Drugs like Viagra and Cialis work by enhancing nitric oxide–mediated vasodilation in the erectile tissues, and studies have shown that they are effective in both men and women.[7]

THE LUNGS

Returning to the anatomy of the upper respiratory system as we descend from the mouth and nose, we arrive at the trachea, or windpipe. The trachea is a rigid tube held open by C-shaped rings made of hard cartilage. This rigidity is essential; without it, the trachea would collapse every time we took a breath. The trachea divides into two bronchi, which split into the right and left lungs. The bronchi continue to divide into bronchioles, and this division happens twenty to twenty-five more times, creating an airway system that looks similar to the roots of a tree. The bronchioles end in saclike structures called alveoli, where the majority of gas exchange takes place.

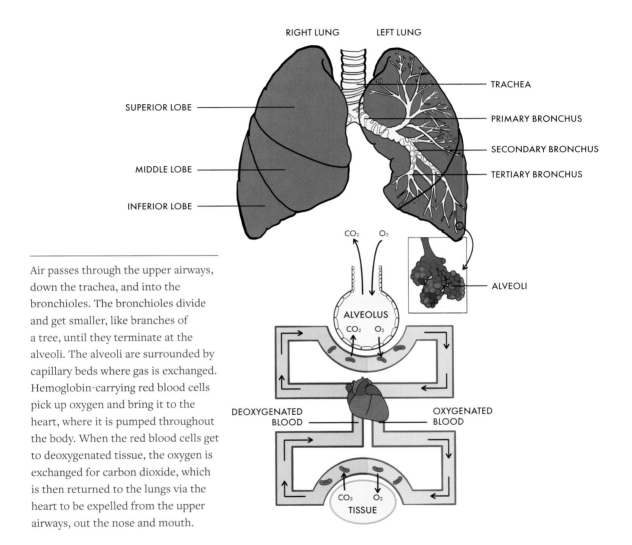

Air passes through the upper airways, down the trachea, and into the bronchioles. The bronchioles divide and get smaller, like branches of a tree, until they terminate at the alveoli. The alveoli are surrounded by capillary beds where gas is exchanged. Hemoglobin-carrying red blood cells pick up oxygen and bring it to the heart, where it is pumped throughout the body. When the red blood cells get to deoxygenated tissue, the oxygen is exchanged for carbon dioxide, which is then returned to the lungs via the heart to be expelled from the upper airways, out the nose and mouth.

Men's lungs hold about 6 liters of air, while the average woman's lungs hold about 4.5 liters. Women's lungs are usually 20 to 25 percent smaller than men's. These values are general, and different textbooks might have different numbers, so please don't get caught up in these values; your lung volume might be completely different. Total lung capacity also depends on a person's age, height, weight, history of smoking, athletic training/conditioning habits, and numerous other factors.

Despite these general numbers, we have the ability to change our vital lung capacity—in other words, how much air we can inhale and how deeply we can exhale. Whether it is possible to stretch lung tissue is a point of contention among researchers, but either way, we can stretch the thoracic cavity that contains the lungs. Think about blowing up a balloon inside a glass jar. The size of the balloon is limited to the size of the jar. Our chest and lungs share a similar relationship. World-record-holding freediver Stig Severinsen's lungs can hold 14 liters,[8] which he attributes to the breathing exercises he does to increase his ability to hold his breath for extended periods.

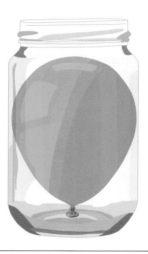

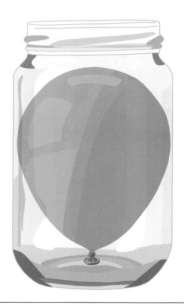

The expansion capability of the lungs is limited to the size of the thoracic cavity. This is similar to blowing up a balloon inside a glass jar. Even if the balloon itself could expand more, its expansion is limited to the size of the jar.

By increasing the size of the jar, we can further expand the balloon. Likewise, to increase our lung capacity, we need to increase the size of our thoracic cavity by stretching our intercostal muscles and strengthening our diaphragm.

The amount of air we displace during normal breathing, or the unconscious breathing we do while at rest, is called tidal volume, and it's usually about one-tenth of total lung capacity, or around 0.5 liter/500 milliliters (mL), which is the average for both men and women. (Men's tidal volume is typically between 550 and 650 mL; for women, it's 450 to 550 mL.) When breathing normally, we breathe from the middle range of our lungs. From the upper limit of our tidal volume to our maximum inhalation is called the inspiratory reserve volume, and this is about 3 liters (3,000 mL). From the lower limit of our tidal volume, where the diaphragm is relaxed, to the maximum forced exhalation is called the expiratory reserve volume, which is about 1.5 liters (1,500 mL). Even after we exhale as much as we can, we still have about 1 liter (1,000 mL) of air left in our lungs; this is called the residual volume. The residual volume keeps the alveolar sacs from collapsing and keeps enough air in the lungs so that the oxygen exchange can happen even after we exhale or while we hold our breath after exhaling.

When we start at the bottom limit of our maximum exhalation and inhale until we reach the top limit of our maximum inhalation, that's called vital lung capacity. Our vital capacity is essentially the total amount of air we can forcefully move in one breath. Vital capacity significantly impacts health, and it's one of the areas that we will focus on improving with the practices in this book. Having a low vital capacity puts us at a higher risk of respiratory disease, and it's directly related to the mortality rate. Our vital capacity naturally decreases with age, but increasing vital capacity has been shown to help slow the aging process.[9]

VO$_2$ MAX

Another marker to gauge fitness, health, and risk of mortality is VO$_2$ max, which stands for volume oxygen maximum. VO$_2$ max is the maximum amount of oxygen that the body can intake and deliver to the muscles during maximum effort. The higher our VO$_2$ max, the better our cardiorespiratory fitness. Having a higher VO$_2$ max makes us better at activities like running, swimming, and biking, and it is an accurate marker for health and mortality.

While most cardio exercises focus on increasing the heart rate, we can improve our VO$_2$ max just through breathing exercises and essentially become better at cardio without doing traditional cardio exercises. I'm not suggesting that you give up cardio exercise and focus only on breathing, but if you also work on the respiratory side of cardiorespiratory fitness, you will increase your endurance, fitness level, and overall health and well-being.

LUNG VOLUMES

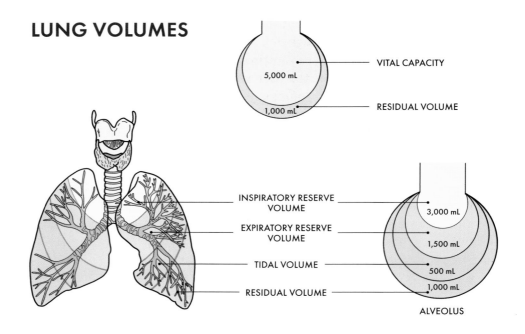

INSPIRATORY RESERVE VOLUME

EXPIRATORY RESERVE VOLUME

TIDAL VOLUME

RESIDUAL VOLUME

VITAL CAPACITY

RESIDUAL VOLUME

5,000 mL

1,000 mL

3,000 mL

1,500 mL

500 mL

1,000 mL

ALVEOLUS

THE MUSCLES OF RESPIRATION

The diaphragm, a thin, dome-shaped muscle that separates the thoracic or chest cavity from the abdominal cavity, is the primary muscle of inhalation and exhalation. The basic mechanics of breathing involve nothing more than simple pressure differentials. To inhale, we reduce the pressure inside our body so that it is less than the atmospheric pressure. The air outside our body rushes into our lungs to equalize the pressures. To exhale, the diaphragm relaxes and returns to its dome shape, which makes the thoracic cavity smaller, increasing the internal pressure and forcing the air out. We find it harder to breathe when we hike in the mountains because the atmospheric pressure is lower at higher altitudes, so we have to work harder to lower our internal pressure.

The diaphragm lowers internal pressure by pulling down or flattening out and expanding the space inside the chest. Through normal tidal volume breathing, the diaphragm does almost all the work, and exhalation is completely passive. The diaphragm relaxes, and the natural tension in the thoracic cavity plus the outside atmospheric pressure aids in an effortless exhale. When we breathe more than our normal tidal volume, we need to recruit our accessory breathing muscles. Increasing the effort to breathe is called forced inhalation or exhalation because inhaling or exhaling requires more force than normal. While the diaphragm still does the majority of the work for inhalation, the external intercostals, serratus anterior, sternocleidomastoid muscle, and scalene muscles assist in lifting the ribs and further expand the chest. The more we open and expand the chest, the lower our inner pressure becomes, and therefore the deeper the inhalation.

RESPIRATORY MUSCLES

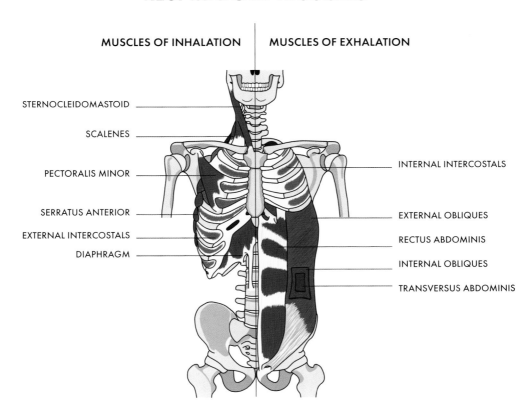

MUSCLES OF INHALATION | MUSCLES OF EXHALATION

STERNOCLEIDOMASTOID

SCALENES

PECTORALIS MINOR

SERRATUS ANTERIOR

EXTERNAL INTERCOSTALS

DIAPHRAGM

INTERNAL INTERCOSTALS

EXTERNAL OBLIQUES

RECTUS ABDOMINIS

INTERNAL OBLIQUES

TRANSVERSUS ABDOMINIS

For forced exhalation, we need to increase the inner pressure in our chest. The diaphragm can aid in exhalation only until it returns to its relaxed dome shape. The intercostal muscles and abdominal muscles do most of the work by pulling the ribs down and making the chest cavity smaller. Really, the abdominis rectus (our six-pack muscles) are the main muscles working.

Many people breathe poorly and insufficiently due to constant engagement of the abdominal muscles, which are our muscles of exhalation. The main reason is that people don't want to let their bellies hang out. I was guilty of this habit for years, and even now, I notice myself unconsciously and unnecessarily engaging my core just because of the habit that formed from vanity and insecurity. Even beyond forced respiration, walking around with our core muscles continuously engaged limits our ability to breathe fully and effortlessly. The core muscles hold the bottom ribs down and belly in, which impedes the diaphragm, in turn forcing the accessory inhale-centric muscles to work harder in order to lift the upper chest and collarbones because we can't expand the bottom ribs or breathe down into the abdominal region. This is known as chest breathing, and it is a tremendous waste of energy, resulting in insufficient shallow breathing. Breathing with the core consistently engaged can also move us into a chronic state of tension and stress that negatively impacts the health and balance of our autonomic nervous system.

You might have heard of diaphragmatic breathing or belly breathing, which refers to breathing with a relaxed core, allowing the stomach to expand. It's a common misconception that when we belly breathe, we are using only our diaphragm, and when we chest breathe, we are using only our accessory chest muscles. Chest breathing doesn't mean that the diaphragm is not functioning. The diaphragm is working in every type of breathing we do. If you've ever had the wind knocked out of you, either from falling flat on your back or being hit in the stomach or solar plexus, you've experienced a temporary paralysis of the diaphragm, and it can feel like you can't breathe or catch your breath. This feeling is what it's like to breathe without using your diaphragm. If you've never had the wind knocked out of you, consider yourself lucky and enjoy the fact that your diaphragm is always working to make breathing as effortless as possible.

CLINICAL VALUES VS. BASELINE VALUES

There is always going to be high variability between what medical textbooks say our normal vital signs should be and the actual numbers in healthy and unhealthy people. For example, a regular pulse rate should be between 60 and 100 beats per minute (bpm). Below 60 bpm is considered bradycardia, or too slow to circulate the blood and deliver oxygen to the cells adequately. My resting heartbeat is around 40 to 45 bpm and drops into the thirties when I do certain breathing exercises or meditation. Most athletes and healthy people have a lower-than-average resting heart rate.

Clinical standards are supposed to be based on the average person. Unfortunately, with the majority of Americans being overweight or obese and sedentary, normal standards don't represent the health-conscious, active population. Clinical baselines give us a starting point, but knowing your baseline vitals and how changes in your heart rate, respiratory rate, blood pressure, and other baselines make you feel is better than any set of numbers you will find in a book. However, if your pulse rate, breathing rate, or blood pressure is *higher* than the clinical average, then it should raise significant concern. I've never met a healthy person whose resting heart rate was over 100 bpm.

When I worked as a paramedic, I used clinical values to evaluate whether a patient was within "normal" limits. If they were outside those limits, I would check if there was a need for immediate intervention. As a paramedic, my concern was life-threatening conditions. I often had patients with resting pulse rates over 150 bpm, but still talking fine and acting normal. The elevated heart rate wasn't going to kill them while they were in the back of my ambulance, so it would be a concern for their doctor to fix. This might be where the problem lies in our modern culture. Things like health and wellness, which should be our responsibility, are not. Instead, we pass our health to other people, like doctors, to "fix." Usually, the fixes do not actually heal us. We mask problems, using pharmaceutical interventions to manipulate conditions such as hypertension (high blood pressure) and tachycardia (rapid heart rate) into "normal" limits, but we never address the real problems, which are easily fixed or prevented by eating better, breathing better, and moving more.

Consider the "normal" clinical numbers as tools, not goals. Your goals should be based on where you are now and working to improve upon that.

The clinical values for a normal breathing rate are twelve to twenty breaths per minute, although the upper limit of twenty breaths per minute is probably over-breathing for a healthy person. Generally, people who are overweight and have a larger body mass have faster and more labored breathing. Most fit, healthy people, especially those with good breathing habits, like nasal breathing with a relaxed belly, breathe between ten and sixteen times per minute. Measuring our breathing rate can be tricky, because as soon as we start thinking about it, we change the way we breathe. When I would take a patient's vital signs, I would pretend to take their pulse while counting the rise and fall of their chest so that I could get an accurate respiration rate.

Again, we move about 500 mL of air during one breath cycle. If we are taking ten breaths per minute, that is the equivalent of breathing 5 liters of air per minute. If our total lung capacity is 6 liters, then our vital capacity, or how much air we can move in one full breath, is around 5 liters, with 1 liter remaining as our residual volume. So why is it important to know how much air we're breathing? I've mentioned some of the disadvantages of over-breathing, but we haven't looked at the many advantages that come from breathing less.

THE BENEFITS OF UNDER-BREATHING

We've already discussed how carbon dioxide increases blood flow and decreases blood pressure by enlarging the blood vessels, improves breathing by opening the bronchioles, and helps the red blood cells with oxygen exchange by changing blood pH (due to the Bohr effect). But isn't it bad to make the blood more acidic? Almost all health professionals preach the value of being more alkaline. Drinking alkaline water and eating a more alkaline diet have been shown to have many health benefits, like lowering inflammation, chronic pain, and the risk of illness and disease. Changing the pH of the blood for any length of time is difficult because of the body's amazing buffering system. Our bodies regulate our blood to remain around a constant pH of 7.4. A sustained change in blood pH is usually the result of a more serious health problem. Although we can mildly change the pH quickly just by breathing fast or slowly, it returns to baseline almost immediately after we resume normal breathing. But the pH of the rest of our bodies' fluids varies a lot more and is significantly affected by the foods we eat. The body is also always looking for homeostasis, which is a state of physiological equilibrium.

Over-breathing temporarily increases blood pH and makes us more alkaline. It also makes us feel hungrier and crave acid-forming foods, like sugars, fats, complex carbohydrates, and processed foods. Generally, over-breathing makes us want the foods that we should limit. The next time you do something that causes you to breathe fast, like sprinting or burpees, notice how hungry you feel afterward and which types of foods you crave. I notice that when I teach all day, I am usually starving later. It's hard to talk for longer periods without over-breathing.

Under-breathing (aka hypoventilation) has the opposite effect. When we breathe less, our blood pH decreases and we become more acidic, which has the effect of suppressing appetite and leads to cravings for more alkaline-forming foods, like fruits and vegetables.

THE EFFECTS OF HYPERVENTILATION VS. HYPOVENTILATION

OVER-BREATHING HYPERVENTILATION		UNDER-BREATHING HYPOVENTILATION	
↓	CARBON DIOXIDE LEVELS	↑	CARBON DIOXIDE LEVELS
↑	BLOOD pH (ALKALINITY)	↓	BLOOD pH (ACIDITY)
	STIMULATES SYMPATHETIC NERVOUS SYSTEM		STIMULATES PARASYMPATHETIC NERVOUS SYSTEM
↑	BRONCHOCONSTRICTION	↑	BRONCHODILATION
↑	VASOCONSTRICTION	↑	VASODILATION
↑	BLOOD PRESSURE	↓	BLOOD PRESSURE
↓	OXYGENATION OF TISSUES (DUE TO BOHR EFFECT)	↑	OXYGENATION OF TISSUES (DUE TO BOHR EFFECT)
↑	TENSION/PAIN	↑	RELAXATION
↑	HUNGER	↓	HUNGER
↑	CRAVINGS FOR ACIDIC-PRODUCING FOOD	↑	CRAVINGS FOR ALKALINE-PRODUCING FOOD
↑	COLONIC TONE	↓	COLONIC TONE

HIGH-ALTITUDE TRAINING EFFECTS FROM BREATHING EXERCISES

My high school was 5,600 feet (1,700 meters) above sea level. Although it was a small school, our wrestling team usually dominated the much larger schools. When teams from other schools would come up the mountain to compete against us, most of our opponents would run out of breath and struggle to keep up because they weren't used to the thinner air. When I wrestled at schools that were closer to sea level, I felt like I had so much more energy and endurance. Training at high elevation boosted our red blood cell count, so we had more oxygen-carrying hemoglobin to supply our muscles, which increased our cardio fitness (VO_2 max) and endurance. We would often win because the other teams were too tired to keep up.

What gave us the advantage over other schools is known as high-altitude training, although most people who do high-altitude training train at much higher elevations, and some endurance athletes even train at elevations higher than 8,000 feet (2,400 meters). Because the air is thinner at higher altitudes and it is harder for the body to deliver oxygen to the cells than it is at sea level, the body makes more red blood cells to keep up with metabolic demands. Many Olympic training centers are located at high elevation to give athletes an advantage.

Lance Armstrong is known as one of the greatest cyclists ever, and he is the only person to have won the Tour de France seven times. However, he was stripped of all his victories after being accused of blood doping. Blood doping involves artificially increasing the number of red blood cells in the bloodstream to boost athletic performance, and some of the methods used can be very dangerous. Most sports have deemed blood doping illegal.

Whether we are training at high altitude or (preferably not) blood doping, having more oxygen-carrying red blood cells increases our athletic performance. As discussed earlier, the body works off of demand. Whatever the body needs, it generates more of; if there is an excess or a lack of need, the body makes less. Chronic over-breathing results in fewer red blood cells, but under-breathing produces more. Breathing less, particularly long breath-holds and breath retention while performing strenuous activities, can simulate high-altitude training and has the same physiological effect. Creating an oxygen-deficient environment and increasing carbon dioxide prompts the body to make more red blood cells to meet our needs, which results in increased cardiorespiratory fitness and endurance levels.

POSTURE AND THE BREATH

Take a breath. If you feel that you are growing taller or your shoulders and collarbones are lifting, then you are likely chest breathing. A natural breath shouldn't be forced; it should be effortless, with little or no noticeable assistance from the accessory breathing muscles, like the intercostals or neck muscles. Even if you take a deep breath, your shoulders and collarbones shouldn't rise; instead, you should feel your rib cage expand outward. Healthy and effective breathing starts with good posture.

One reason poor posture is so bad for us is that it significantly impairs the diaphragm's ability to function properly. Think of a drum head (the part you strike to make noise). It sounds best when it is pulled uniformly taut. If you squeeze the opening of the drum, then you will warp the drum head, and the drumming will sound awful. The diaphragm is similar; it works best when it is equally taut, as it naturally is when we have good posture. When we slouch forward and roll our shoulders in, the chest compresses and the sternum and rib cage have trouble expanding. The diaphragm isn't able to contract properly and pull down to expand our chest as we inhale. Poor posture leads to compensatory breathing patterns, like lifting the shoulders and collarbones, which can lead to chronic back pain. These types of compensatory breathing patterns also stimulate the nervous system's stress responses that can create feelings of anxiety and depression.

ACTION OF RESPIRATION

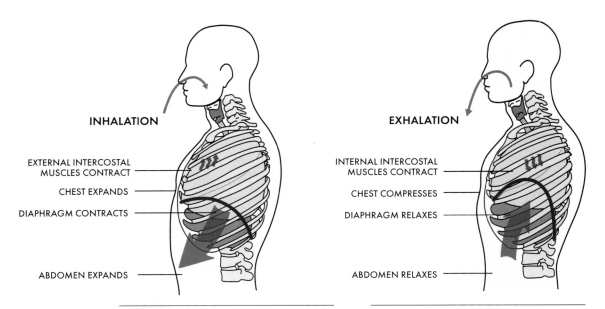

INHALATION

EXTERNAL INTERCOSTAL MUSCLES CONTRACT

CHEST EXPANDS

DIAPHRAGM CONTRACTS

ABDOMEN EXPANDS

EXHALATION

INTERNAL INTERCOSTAL MUSCLES CONTRACT

CHEST COMPRESSES

DIAPHRAGM RELAXES

ABDOMEN RELAXES

The diaphragm is a dome-shaped muscle. As we inhale, the diaphragm contracts, moving downward and flattening out. This action, along with the lift of the external intercostal muscles and expansion of the abdomen, increases the thoracic cavity's size and pulls air into the lungs.

During an exhalation, the diaphragm passively relaxes, returning to its dome shape. The intercostal muscles move the ribs down, and the abdomen relaxes, decreasing the thoracic cavity's size and expelling the air from the lungs.

For proper posture, whether sitting or standing, the spine should maintain its natural curves. The lower lumbar spine should have a mild lordotic or inward-curving shape. The upper thoracic spine should have a mild kyphotic or outward-curving shape, and the neck should have a natural lordotic curve where the head is not extending forward. The shoulders should be slightly forward in a neutral position and not pulled back like a soldier's when standing at attention. The pelvis should be tilted slightly forward while sitting and neutral while standing.

Let's talk about chairs since we are talking about posture. Most chairs place us back in the seat against the backrest. The front of the chair is higher than the back of the chair, and the knees are higher than the hips. While sitting like this might be comfortable because it takes little effort, it's a significant contributor to low back pain and major back problems, weak core stabilizing muscles, and poor breathing patterns. We should sit in chairs that are flat and firm and don't cause us to rock back into the seat. For any chairs you have that aren't like this, I suggest getting a cushion that elevates your hips higher than your knees, especially in your car. The best place to sit is on the floor, preferably with a little cushion to elevate your hips so that you can naturally align your spine. Sitting should be active and take a little bit of effort to maintain. You know you are sitting right when you feel a need to get up and walk around every thirty minutes or so.

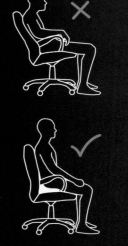

With good posture, completely relax and soften your stomach. Did you notice how much you were holding it in and how much it expanded? If you didn't notice any change, good job—one less thing to fix. To fully relax the stomach can be very challenging for most people, especially athletes, because we tend to hold in our bellies the most. I work with many athletic people, and when I train them to relax the stomach completely, most of them physically can't, not because the core is so strong but because they've been subconsciously holding it in for so many years that they don't know how to fully relax their core muscles. It took me some practice to be able to do it myself, and I still catch myself unnecessarily holding in my belly. You know your stomach is relaxed if it is soft and you can push four fingers into your abs, toward your spine, with relatively little resistance. Your belly should also bounce back to the resting position without delay. If it doesn't immediately spring back, you are still engaging your core muscles. When you're able to master relaxing your core, you'll be able to breathe more effectively, and you'll also increase your vital capacity. When you assume good posture and relax your belly, proper, efficient breathing should happen naturally.

To put it all together, stand or sit upright so that your spine maintains its natural curvature. Relax your shoulders and release all muscle engagement of your core, especially the rectus abdominis muscles. Relax your jaw and face. Slowly inhale through your nose. Allow the breath to move down toward your belly and the rib cage to expand outward. It should feel like your chest has expanded 360 degrees into your back as well. When the rib cage lifts, your shoulders and collarbones should remain in place. The intercostal muscles that elevate the ribs pull upward toward your collarbones but shouldn't lift them. The exhalation should be totally passive, meaning without effort or muscular engagement, as the diaphragm returns to its neutral position.

Pause at the top of the inhalation and at the bottom of the exhalation. A great way to slow your breathing is to practice lengthening these pauses. Also, a slower inhalation brings in more nitric oxide. The exhalation should be slightly longer than the inhalation. Count your respiration cycle and aim to slow it to ten to twelve breaths per minute. If breathing that slowly feels natural, then work on slowing it down even more. If twelve breaths per minute is a struggle to maintain, breathe slightly slower than what feels comfortable. Consciously breathe like this for fifteen to thirty minutes a day or whenever you think about it, until you have created a new habit of breathing properly. Breathing is life; if we want to be healthy, we need to learn how to breathe well.

NOTES

[1]John A. Kellum, "Determinants of blood pH in health and disease," *Critical Care* 4, no. 1 (2000): 6–14, doi:10.1186/cc644.

[2]A. K. Patel, A. Benner, and J. S. Cooper, "Physiology, Bohr effect." [Updated 2019 Jul 29]. In: *StatPearls* [Internet]. Treasure Island (FL): StatPearls Publishing; 2020 Jan–. Available from: https://www.ncbi.nlm.nih.gov/books/NBK526028/.

[3]Roni Kahana-Zweig, Maya Geva-Sagiv, Aharon Weissbrod, Lavi Secundo, Nachum Soroker, and Noam Sobel, "Measuring and characterizing the human nasal cycle," *PloS One* 11, no. 10 (2016): e0162918, doi:10.1371/journal.pone.0162918.

[4]Andreas K. Nussler and Timothy R. Billiar, "Inflammation, immunoregulation, and inducible nitric oxide synthase," *Journal of Leukocyte Biology* 54, no. 2 (1993): 171–8.

[5]Genef C. Ribeiro, Isadora D. Dos Santos, Ana C. Santos, Luiz R. Paranhos, and Carla P. César, "Influence of the breathing pattern on the learning process: a systematic review of literature," *Brazil Journal of Otorhinolaryngology* 82, no. 4 (2016): 466–78, doi:10.1016/j.bjorl.2015.08.026.

[6]Victor Dishy, Gbenga Sofowora, Paul A. Harris, Michelle Kandcer, Frank Zhan, Alastair J. J. Wood, and C. Michael Stein, "The effect of sildenafil on nitric oxide-mediated vasodilation in healthy men," *Clinical Pharmacology & Therapeutics* 70, no. 3 (2001): 270–9, doi:10.1067/mcp.2001.117995.

[7]Kyan J. Allahdadi, Rita C. A. Tostes, and R. Clinton Webb, "Female sexual dysfunction: therapeutic options and experimental challenges," *Cardiovascular & Hematological Agents in Medicinal Chemistry* 7, no. 4 (2009): 260–9, doi:10.2174/187152509789541882.

[8]Kevin Lynch, "Stig Severinsen sets world record double with pair of daring freedives beneath the ice," Guinness World Records, October 16, 2013, available from: https://www.guinnessworldrecords.com/news/2013/10/freediver-stig-severinsen-sets-new-world-record-with-swim-250-feet-below-the-ice-on-a-single-breath-52227/.

[9]Erin M. Lowery, Aleah L. Brubaker, Erica Kuhlmann, and Elizabeth J. Kovacs, "The aging lung," *Clinical Interventions in Aging* 8 (2013): 1489–96, doi:10.2147/CIA.S51152.

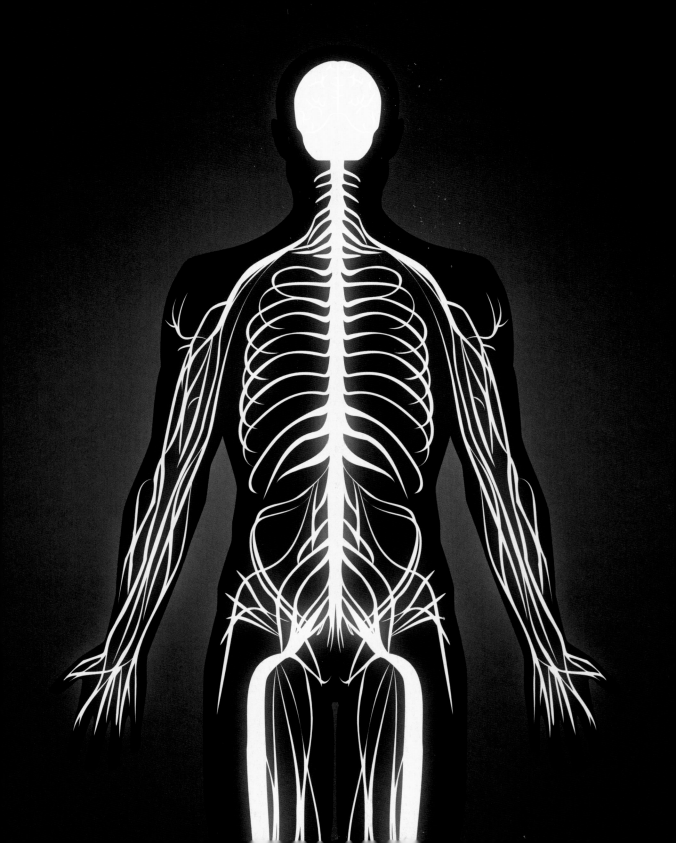

[SECTION 2]
SYSTEMS OF BALANCE

Our bodies are continuously regulating our blood pressure, heart rate, internal temperature, pH levels, organ functions, fluid levels, digestive functions, and numerous other physiological properties to maintain a vital state of balance. They do this regulating without thought or external input. In fact, they automatically regulate so many things that it would be impossible for us to consciously regulate any one of them for twenty-four hours without developing severe health problems or dying. Imagine having to tell your heart to beat every single time, or instruct your kidneys when and how much blood to filter and turn into urine so that you don't poison yourself with the toxins your body created or become overly dehydrated from filtering too much blood.

Luckily for us, we have systems in place that maintain balance automatically. If you're not already aware of how the autonomic nervous system functions, don't worry—we're going to cover it in great detail! What you might not be attuned to is how these functions link directly to our emotions. As we undergo emotional changes, we have corresponding physiological changes. This link is clearly seen in the detrimental impact that stress has on us physically. What affects the mind affects the body and vice versa.

While we can't control most of our bodily functions, which is probably a good thing, we can control the breath. The breath is automatic but also consciously controlled. We can use the breath as a tool to affect all the physiological systems that we can't consciously control otherwise. Because our mood and emotional state also correspond to our autonomic nervous system, we can use the breath here to help us control how we feel and how we interact with ourselves and others.

Understanding the autonomic nervous system's function creates a map that lays out our physical and emotional topography. Knowing how the breath directly impacts the autonomic nervous system allows us to navigate toward our goals. The autonomic nervous system is one of many "systems of balance" that we can use to navigate the mind and body. In this section, we will look at five different systems of balance and the hypothetical maps they create to help guide us to physical and emotional harmony. While each "map" or system might appear different, they all reference the same thing: our holistic self. Just like looking at various maps of a city, one may show the roadways, one the topography, and another the utility lines, but all these maps overlay the same city, and moving north on one map takes you north across all maps. In the same regard, all the systems of balance are intrinsically linked.

We'll begin with the first two "systems of balance," which are really one, but two different ways of looking at the same thing.

THE AUTONOMIC NERVOUS SYSTEM AND THE POLYVAGAL THEORY

The human nervous system consists of two main parts:

- **The central nervous system** includes the brain and spinal cord.
- **The peripheral nervous system** comprises the nerves that leave or return to the brain or spinal cord.

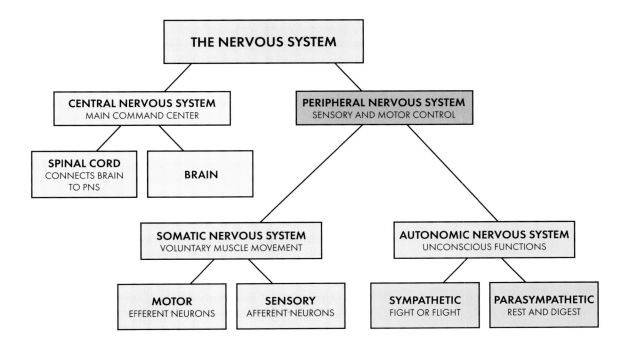

The central nervous system is responsible for analyzing all incoming information and stimulation from the body. After deciphering those messages, it sends a response along the peripheral nervous system to the appropriate area in the body. Most of the information we take in goes directly to the brain for decoding via afferent (incoming) sensory neurons. Then the brain sends out an action signal via the efferent (outgoing) motor neurons. If the stimulus requires an immediate response, like stepping on a nail or touching a hot pan, the response is dealt with at the spinal cord, and the signal never reaches the brain. The spinal cord senses information like "hot" or "sharp" and sends a message via the motor neurons, creating an instant reflex loop that tells the appropriate body part to move. This reaction is known as the reflex arc.

The peripheral nervous system branches again into the somatic nervous system and the autonomic nervous system.

- **The somatic nervous system** has two main functions. The first is sensory. It communicates along the afferent pathways, bringing information back to the central nervous system from our sense organs using various types of sensory receptors. Mechanoreceptors detect changes in pressure, thermoreceptors gauge changes in temperature, and nociceptors sense pain. The somatic nervous system also brings information from our senses of sight, taste, smell, hearing, and equilibrium and then sends the brain a message that paints a picture of our outer and inner worlds. The second function is to carry signals from the central nervous system along efferent neural pathways to our skeletal muscles for controlled movement.

- **The autonomic nervous system** communicates with our organs and glands. It is responsible for regulating all involuntary and unconscious functions of the body, like digestion, maintaining blood pressure, regulating heart rate, and incognizant breathing. An easy way to think of it is that the somatic nervous system relays all thinking actions, whereas the autonomic nervous system is for nonthinking functions.

The autonomic nervous system divides again into the sympathetic and parasympathetic pathways. Although these two pathways are mostly antagonistic, they are meant to function concertedly to maintain the regularity of involuntary functions. Changes in our physical, mental, or emotional condition dictate which pathway is dominant.

- **The sympathetic nervous system** is known as the fight-or-flight response, meaning it is more active in response to stressful situations.

- **The parasympathetic nervous system,** also known as "rest and digest," is more engaged when we are in relaxed states such as sleeping and eating. It is also vital for sexual organ function.

With terms like "fight or flight" and "rest and digest," it's easy to think that these two pathways oppose each other, as though one is always fighting for dominance. But in reality, they mostly work with each other in contrast to maintain homeostasis throughout our bodily functions. What I mean by working "in contrast" is that the difference between the two helps bring out the aspects of the opposing pathway—like adding black to a painting brings out the brightness of white and the vibrancy of colors. The autonomic nervous system, through contrasting stimulation or regression of the sympathetic or parasympathetic nervous system, helps increase the opposing effects to maintain homeostasis. The acute sympathetic response is there for times of extreme danger, but most of the time, we are neither fighting nor running for our lives. Neither are we sleeping or digesting. We are most often somewhere between these two states.

I've heard and read many explanations that the two systems function like a switch: when one is on, the other is off. When we are in a highly stressed state, this might be true, but the body is much more intelligent and complicated than "one is on, and the other is off." In activities such as sexual arousal and ejaculation, the sympathetic, parasympathetic, and somatic nervous systems are all active. If the primary function of these two systems is to regulate the balance of life-providing functions like pumping blood, controlling blood pressure, regulating hormone secretion, and digesting food, then the on/off analogy doesn't make sense.

A better way of understanding the cooperative roles between the sympathetic and parasympathetic nervous systems is to think of them as hot and cold faucets. When both systems are functioning correctly and one isn't overstimulated, the water is nice and warm. This balance of the two functioning systems is called autonomic tone. As the situation dictates, more hot or cold water can be added, and when needed, the water can be all hot or all cold. In reality, though, there is no switch or faucet. Both systems are functioning, releasing hormones and neurotransmitters, titrated as needed throughout the body to handle whatever situation we are experiencing dynamically.

Imagine you are asleep in bed, and then all of a sudden, a loud beeping noise wakes you. The smell of smoke fills the room. In an instant, you are completely alert and super focused. Your house is on fire, and you need to get out! Your heart starts racing, your pupils dilate, your blood vessels constrict to push more blood into your muscles, and your breathing becomes shallow and rapid. Now, imagine you're getting ready to give a big speech to hundreds of people, and you have no idea what you're going to say. As you walk onto the stage, you feel a tightness in your chest as your heart starts beating faster and your mouth feels dry. You freeze, unable to think, move, or speak. One more scenario: you're watching a horror movie, and the main character is hiding under the bed as the killer enters the room. You feel anxious; you start sweating even though it's not hot in the room, and you even begin to hyperventilate.

These three situations are all very different. In the first scenario, you are in real danger, and your sympathetic nervous system responds precisely how it is supposed to. But in the other two situations, there is no actual danger, yet because your mind perceives the situations as dangerous, you have a sympathetic fight-or-flight response. It's important to recognize that actual and perceived danger elicit the same reaction. And although these are examples of a more extreme response, in our busy society, the majority of people live in a constant state of stress and anxiety. This chronic stimulation of the sympathetic nervous system leads to major cardiac and respiratory illnesses, digestive issues, and other health problems.

Because so many people deal with chronic stress and, therefore, are in chronic sympathetic activation, the sympathetic nervous system is discussed in a negative way, and probably for good reason. Most people need to learn how to decrease chronic stress and increase parasympathetic tone to bring balance. But there is another way to look at the sympathetic nervous system, and that is activation and mobilization. When we wake from sleep, sympathetic tone increases. The shift in tone is minor, but we need this activation to get going. Often we try to aid it by drinking coffee because we are not getting enough rest to restore our baseline. The more activity we do, the more the sympathetic nervous system works to give us the energy we need. When we start to slow down, the parasympathetic nervous system slowly applies the brakes, and this harmonious relationship continues to support our lifestyle and needs.

The sympathetic nervous system originates in the thoracic and lumbar regions of the spine. Preganglionic nerves exit the spine and connect to the sympathetic chain of ganglion, which are located near the spine. From here, postganglionic nerve fibers travel to organs, blood vessels, and glands. The postganglionic fibers are myelinated, which enables them to send the signal much faster than unmyelinated preganglionic fibers; this allows the signal to travel to the organs much quicker than it does in the parasympathetic nervous system, where the unmyelinated preganglionic nerves are much longer because the parasympathetic ganglia are located near or within the target organs. This myelination allows for a quicker sympathetic response. The sympathetic nervous system functions primarily to react quickly to perceived danger or potential threats—i.e., fight or flight. So the bodily response is to mobilize immediately. The pupils dilate so we can see more, the heart beats faster, and the blood vessels constrict to increase muscle perfusion. The bronchi in the lungs open up so we can breathe better, the adrenal glands release adrenaline, giving us a rush of energy, and urinary and digestive functions are inhibited.

The parasympathetic nervous system (*para* meaning "around") originates above and below the sympathetic nervous system, in the skull and sacrum. From the brain stem, cranial nerves III, VII, and IX travel to the eyes, face, and mouth, controlling constriction of the pupils, salivation, and lacrimation (the flow of tears). Cranial nerve X, known as the vagus nerve, travels to the majority of the abdominal organs and viscera. The vagus nerve is the most significant component of the sympathetic nervous system. It's responsible for slowing the heart rate and contractility, tightening the airways in the lungs, moving food down the digestive tract, limiting inflammation, and helping the immune system. From the sacrum, parasympathetic fibers connect to the kidneys, bladder, and sexual organs. The parasympathetic nervous system physically functions to aid in rest and recovery, digestion and excretion, and reproduction. The autonomic nervous system's function and influence are significant when it comes to social engagement, mood, and outlook on life.

THE AUTONOMIC NERVOUS SYSTEM

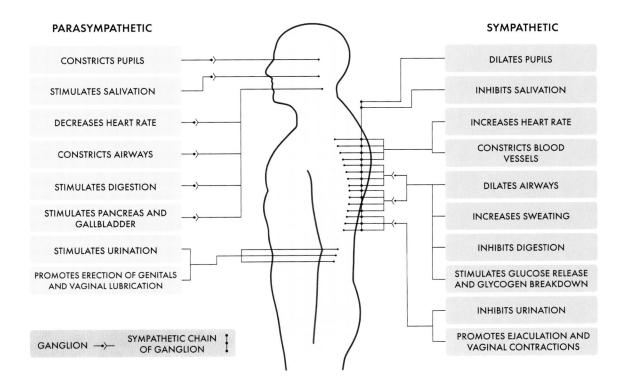

Dr. Stephen Porges developed the polyvagal theory based on the two branches of the vagus nerve that control most of the parasympathetic nervous system: the ventral vagal complex and the dorsal vagal complex. His approach divides the autonomic nervous system into a three-part system consisting of the ventral vagal complex, sympathetic nervous system, and dorsal vagal complex.[1]

Although the ventral vagal and dorsal vagal complexes both stem from the vagus nerve, they function and respond very differently.

- The dorsal vagal complex is responsible for most digestive functions and regulates the organs below the diaphragm. It is the older primal evolutionary branch and is responsible for our earliest stress response, also known as the "freeze" response. In situations involving a high degree of fear, overstimulation of the dorsal vagal complex can lock us up, rendering us unable to move or act, as we see in many reptiles and some mammals reacting to extreme danger. When the dorsal vagal complex is in dysfunction, we become withdrawn and antisocial. Increasing the dorsal vagal complex tone calmly and peacefully—i.e., not under danger or stress—brings us into a state of deep relaxation, as we experience in meditation.

- The ventral vagal complex regulates the functions of the heart and the respiratory system. It is associated with social engagement and is most dominant when we are healthy and happy.

The polyvagal theory expresses the reactive relationship of the autonomic nervous system in a hierarchical order of safety or danger. The ventral vagal complex, at the top of the system, is related to how we conduct ourselves in a positive manner around others; interact with our friends, family, and strangers; and present ourselves in social situations. If we sense danger or a threat, then the sympathetic nervous system reacts with the fight-or-flight response. If the situation is perceived as life-threatening, then the dorsal vagal complex reacts with immobilization, dissociation, and shock. If we are in a place where we feel safe, then stimulation of the sympathetic nervous system moves us toward a healthy state of mobilization where we can work, dance, play, do sports, and physically interact. The dorsal vagal complex adds balance by bringing us into a state of rest, rejuvenation, and deep relaxation.

In this model, we see the mutable interactions of the autonomic nervous system and the importance of each part's function concerning a healthy and safe state versus reacting to a threat or danger.

THE POLYVAGAL THEORY

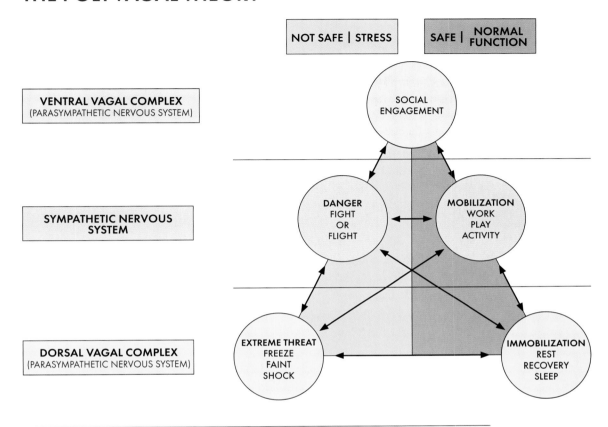

The parasympathetic nervous system is controlled primarily by the vagus nerve, which has two branches: the ventral vagal complex (VVC) and the dorsal vagal complex (DVC). These two branches, combined with the sympathetic nervous system (SNS), make up the autonomic nervous system (ANS) under the polyvagal theory.

The polyvagal theory maps out the response of the ANS when stimulated while feeling safe or feeling stress or danger. In a healthy state of balance, we are primarily stimulating the VVC. When we experience changes from external or internal stimuli, we can quickly shift from safe to unsafe or vice versa and switch branches of the ANS. We can also get "stuck" in the SNS or DVC if we remain in a chronic state of stress.

HEART RATE VARIABILITY

So how do you know that your nervous system is balanced and regulated? Probably the best way is just to observe yourself:

- Do you usually feel stressed or overwhelmed?

- How many hours do you sleep each night?

- How would you rate the quality of your sleep?

- Do you get sick easily or often?

- When you are sick, how long does it typically take you to recover?

- Do you exercise regularly?

It's easy to know that your nervous system is out of balance if your answers to these questions are not what you'd like them to be. But you can have a low-stress life, sleep well, and rarely get sick and still not have a healthy regulation of your nervous system.

One of the tools used to understand the health of the nervous system is heart rate variability, or HRV. Heart rate variability is a measurement of the distance between heartbeats in milliseconds. If your heart beats sixty times per minute, it isn't necessarily beating once every second; it is beating an *average* of once per second. As we breathe in and out, the duration of each heartbeat changes. This fluctuation exists because inhalations stimulate our sympathetic nervous system; in turn, the sympathetic nervous system speeds up our heart and makes it beat at a more regular and consistent tempo. However, our exhalations stimulate the parasympathetic nervous system, which causes our heart rate to slow down and our heart rhythm to become more irregular, as though to "breathe" with our respirations, which again is a positive sign of a healthy autonomic nervous system and increased parasympathetic tone.

HRV is a marker of the health of the autonomic nervous system, revealing the relationship between the sympathetic and parasympathetic nervous systems. The lower the HRV number (the more regular and consistent the heartbeat), the more dominant the sympathetic tone is. The higher the HRV number, the less sympathetic tone.[2] Essentially, our heart breathes along with our breath, which directly affects the nervous system. The higher the variability, the healthier the state of your nervous system.

Because we can make our autonomic nervous system respond by speeding up, slowing down, or changing the depth of our inhales and exhales, our HRV score is only a reliable measurement of the health of our nervous system when it's taken while we're asleep. However, it is good to monitor how our breath practices are increasing our HRV in real time. Doing breath practices that increase HRV has long-lasting effects, and, in addition to good sleep and low stress, breathing is one of the best ways to regulate nervous system function.

High HRV shows more than just the balance of the autonomic nervous system. It's also an excellent indication of cardiovascular health, the ability to handle stress and exercise, and a high fitness level. People with high HRV also generally have strong willpower, a calm demeanor, good social engagement, and self-control. Low HRV is related to chronic stress, pain, inflammation, depression, and increased risk of cardiovascular disease, cancer, and death.

HEART RATE VARIABILITY

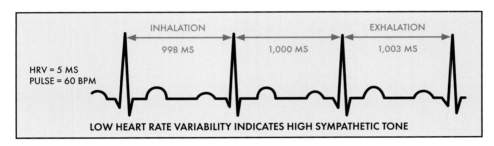

INHALATION — 998 MS — 1,000 MS — EXHALATION — 1,003 MS

HRV = 5 MS
PULSE = 60 BPM

LOW HEART RATE VARIABILITY INDICATES HIGH SYMPATHETIC TONE

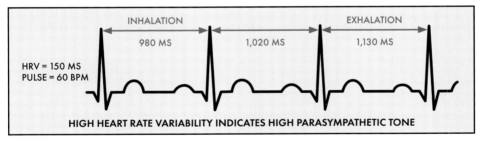

INHALATION — 980 MS — 1,020 MS — EXHALATION — 1,130 MS

HRV = 150 MS
PULSE = 60 BPM

HIGH HEART RATE VARIABILITY INDICATES HIGH PARASYMPATHETIC TONE

Heart rate variability is one of the best ways to measure the health of the autonomic nervous system. HRV measures the time between heartbeats to determine the rate of variability. Low HRV (less variability between heartbeats) can result from high levels of stress from either internal or external stimuli; increased stimulation of the sympathetic nervous system (fight or flight); poor sleep, diet, or fitness; alcohol consumption; illness; and inadequate rest or recovery after exercise. Higher HRV (more variability between heartbeats) is a good indicator of a healthy autonomic nervous system; low stress; good sleep, diet, and fitness; a healthy immune system; and adequate rest and recovery after exercise.

MEASURING AND IMPROVING
HEART RATE VARIABILITY

When I learned about the importance of HRV, I went out and bought a monitor. There are several good products out there. The most accurate for measuring real-time HRV are chest straps that link to an app. In the beginning, I used one to see the real-time effects of my various breathing exercises. Now, I wear a smart ring when I sleep to monitor my HRV, my sleep cycles and durations, and my resting heart rate, along with a few other health markers, so I can make lifestyle changes that make me feel better and healthier.

I consider myself to be very healthy and fit, my outlook on life is positive, and I rarely feel stressed. But when I started checking my HRV, I was shocked at how low it was.

Average healthy HRV decreases rapidly with age and can vary significantly between people of the same age. It's best not to compare yourself to others or think that you should achieve a certain score. Because my HRV was lower than I thought it should be, I thought I had serious problems when I compared mine to my friend who is ten years younger. The average HRV of someone around twenty-five years old is between 55 and 100 milliseconds (ms); at forty, HRV is 35 to 65 ms; and in someone over fifty-five, HRV drops to 25 to 45 ms. But these numbers still vary significantly regardless of age and health condition, and you shouldn't give it too much thought if yours is below the average for your age. Knowing your baseline is more important than knowing the average HRV score for your age and trying to get your HRV to a certain score. When you start monitoring your HRV, it will take you a few weeks to find your baseline. Once you understand where you usually are, it will be easy to see how little things can have a significant impact and what you can change to improve your health.

My HRV was low mainly due to my lifestyle. As a traveling yoga teacher, I fly all over the world, and I regularly deal with jet lag and poor sleep. The other thing that was killing me was over-breathing. I never thought of myself as an over-breather, but on average, I talk for more than twenty hours every weekend, either lecturing or teaching, and this increases considerably when I lead teacher trainings.

While I still teach just as much, if not more, am always traveling, and am regularly jet-lagged, I've been able to improve my score considerably. Because my two biggest problems were lack of sleep and over-breathing, those were the first two things I worked on rectifying. I did as much as I could for sleep, such as not drinking coffee after noon, limiting alcohol consumption, reducing exposure to blue light, and going to bed earlier. I also started to do much more *pranayama* (see Section 3), and I began to do breathing exercises specifically to increase my HRV and restore the balance of my autonomic nervous system (see the Equanimity breath sequence on pages 180 to 184). These practices dramatically improved my HRV, my quality of sleep, and the time it took me to recover from jet lag.

It takes several weeks of monitoring your HRV to understand how the lifestyle changes you make will affect your score. HRV is a real-time tool to track the effects of things like diet, sleep, stress, and exercise, and it can vary from day to day. Sometimes I wake up feeling tired and fatigued, and I know my HRV will be low before even looking at it. So I take it easy, maybe skip my handstands for the day or do a more relaxed yoga practice or something more restorative, like meditation. Low HRV can be a sign that you haven't fully recovered, and you need rest. Other times I feel fine, but my HRV is really low. I've found that when my HRV is low and I decide to push it, I end up having a poor practice, getting sick, or even injured.

Many, if not all, of the breathing exercises in this book will help improve your HRV and the health and balance of your autonomic nervous system, even if that is not the specific intention of a particular exercise.

THE POLYVAGAL THEORY AND THE IMPORTANCE OF FEELING SAFE

The autonomic nervous system reacts directly to emotion, stress, and how we are breathing. When our perception of our environment switches from feeling safe to feeling scared or anxious, the stress response generates changes in our breathing pattern. If we reverse the reaction by changing our breathing patterns, we can also change the response of our autonomic nervous system, our associated emotions, and possibly our perception of the environment. Hopefully, we are not living in a continuous state of stress and fear and do not find ourselves often needing to use the breath to bring us back to a relaxed state.

The polyvagal theory emphasizes the importance of how the autonomic nervous system is stimulated. It makes a clear distinction between how the nervous system reacts if we are feeling safe and how it reacts if we are feeling afraid or threatened. Feeling unsafe stimulates the sympathetic nervous system and triggers the fight-or-flight response. If the fear is overly intense or the situation seems life-threatening, then the freeze response that is associated with the dorsal vagal complex of the parasympathetic nervous system is triggered.

In contrast, when we feel safe in our environment and activate the sympathetic nervous system, we move toward a mobilization response, where energy to be active, work, play, and socialize is increased. Even though it is still the sympathetic nervous system being activated, its effect on our emotions and physiology is very different. The same is true when we feel safe in a relaxed state and move into the dorsal vagal complex: we enter into a state where we can rest, repair, digest, meditate, and sleep, as discussed earlier.

The third part of the autonomic nervous system and the other branch of the vagus nerve that is a part of the parasympathetic nervous system is the ventral vagal complex. The ventral vagal complex, also known as the social engagement branch, is most active when we feel safe and balanced. It also helps us correlate our breathing patterns and responses with the other energetic systems, such as the *nadis, gunas,* and *prana vayus,* which we'll discover in the next section.

I reiterate the roles of the autonomic nervous system now because as you learn how to use the breath to stimulate the autonomic nervous system, it's vital to practice from a place of feeling safe. Some of the exercises that we will do later on in the book can incite anxiety or panic attacks because the rapid breathing patterns are similar to the reactionary breathing patterns that people have during such attacks. Revisiting similar breathing patterns can cause the trauma or feelings that triggered those breathing patterns to resurface. But the same practices that can prompt a panic attack can also help you never have an attack again. The goal is to train yourself to feel safe while doing these types of breathing exercises so that the psychophysiological responses associated with them will ultimately fade.

As explained in more detail in Section 3, the breath can be divided into four parts: the inhalation, inner breath retention, exhalation, and outer breath retention. Each component of the breath has a direct physiological effect on the autonomic nervous system. The inhalation activates the sympathetic nervous system, which manifests as an increased heart rate. Making the breath quicker and deeper also stimulates a more sympathetic tone. In turn, exhaling stimulates the parasympathetic nervous system, as evidenced by a decreased heart rate. Slowing the breath down, especially on the exhale, stimulates an even more parasympathetic tone.

BREATH EXERCISES FOR STIMULATING THE AUTONOMIC NERVOUS SYSTEM

These next six breathing exercises explore how changing the breath, either by speeding it up, slowing it down, or breathing deeper or shallower, has an immediate effect on our nervous system and, in turn, our energy levels and emotional state. Each component of the breath is linked to our nervous system; therefore, we can stimulate or balance the autonomic nervous system as we see from the direct influence on our heart rate variability. These exercises can be used to quickly change our mood and energy levels as needed. Each breathing technique is simple and can be done at any time, anywhere. Sections 4 and 5 go into more involved and effective ways to use the breath to influence our wants and needs directly.

EXERCISE 1: INCREASING SYMPATHETIC TONE

Take a few moments to breathe naturally and notice your energy level. When you feel ready, inhale fully and quickly through your nose for three to four seconds. After you fill your lungs, open your mouth and sigh to release the breath. Make sure the exhalation is quicker than the inhalation. Continue for thirty seconds to a minute. Afterward, let your breath return to normal and take a few moments to notice if your energy levels have changed. You should feel a little more energized. If you practice this breath longer, you'll feel a more significant response.

EXERCISE 2: INCREASING PARASYMPATHETIC TONE

Take a few moments to breathe naturally and notice your energy level; it's okay if you are still feeling energized from the first exercise. Take a slow, moderate inhale through your nose for five to seven seconds. Slowly exhale through your nose for ten to fourteen seconds. Continue for thirty seconds to a minute. Take a few moments to notice any differences. You should feel more relaxed. Doubling the length of the exhalation and slowing the breath stimulates a more parasympathetic tone, which slows the heart rate and lowers blood pressure.

EXERCISE 3: BALANCING THE AUTONOMIC NERVOUS SYSTEM

Take a few moments to breathe naturally and notice your energy level. If you are feeling low on energy, do exercise 1 until you start to feel your energy levels rise. If you feel very energetic or anxious, do exercise 2 until you begin to feel your nervous energy diminish. Once you approach your baseline, inhale through your nose for eight to ten seconds, take a comfortable pause at the top of the inhalation, and then exhale through your nose for eight to ten seconds. Repeat for one to two minutes to feel the desired effect. Matching the in-breath and the out-breath while also slowing the breath helps regulate the autonomic nervous system and bring us into a more balanced state, stimulating the ventral vagal complex.

Breath retention stimulates the autonomic nervous system in different ways depending on the intensity of the breath-hold, our level of training, and how comfortable we feel while holding our breath. Adding breath retention after an inhalation or exhalation increases carbon dioxide levels, which stimulates the parasympathetic nervous system. Increasing carbon dioxide levels also facilitates increased oxygen delivery to the cells, and improved cellular respiration increases energy levels. Breath retention after an inhalation brings us into the ventral vagal complex, leaving us feeling more balanced, and, if paired with breathing that focuses on inhalations, results in more balanced energy. Holding our breath after an exhalation brings us into the dorsal vagal tone, and we generally feel much more relaxed in ways akin to rest-and-digest.

Breath retention with empty lungs is much more challenging because we have only 1,000 to 1,200 mL of residual air in our lungs for gas exchange, making the need to breathe feel much more urgent. This urgency can quickly evoke panic and activate the sympathetic nervous system, stimulating the fight-or-flight response, which is never the response we want when doing any type of breathing exercise.

EXERCISE 4: INCREASING BALANCED SYMPATHETIC TONE WITH BREATH RETENTION

Take a moment to establish your baseline. Take a full, deep breath through your nose over three to four seconds. Hold your breath at the top of the inhalation for fifteen seconds. Open your mouth and exhale quickly with a sigh. Repeat for one to two minutes. Pause for a moment to feel the effects of the practice. This exercise should leave you feeling more balanced and energized with less of an anxious sensation than you might have experienced in exercise 1. This is because both the sympathetic nervous system and the ventral vagal complex are being stimulated. Try doing exercise 1 and exercise 4 back-to-back to see how the two slightly different practices affect you.

EXERCISE 5: INCREASING PARASYMPATHETIC TONE WITH BREATH RETENTION

Breathe calmly for a few moments. Inhale slowly for five to seven seconds. Exhale for ten to fourteen seconds, and then hold your breath after the exhalation for another ten to fourteen seconds. Repeat for thirty seconds to a minute. Allow your breath to return to normal and notice the effects of the practice. You may have had two very different responses. If the breath retention was easy for you, the effect might be a deep sense of calm; if it was challenging, it might result in anxiety or agitation. With practice, you can maintain a relaxed state and parasympathetic tone, even adding breath retention after the exhalation where you feel extremely challenged.

EXERCISE 6: BOX BREATHING

This exercise focuses on creating equal lengths through all four parts of the breath. Inhale for a count of five. Hold your breath after the inhalation for a count of five. Exhale for a count of five. Hold your breath after the exhalation for a count of five. Repeat for five to ten rounds. This exercise is great for balancing the autonomic nervous system and stimulating ventral vagal tone, resulting in a balanced, equanimous state. This technique is known as equal ratio breathing, and we'll explore it in greater detail in Section 3 (see pages 114 to 117).

The autonomic nervous system and its counterpart, the polyvagal theory, establish how the body regulates, balances, or shifts energy as we look at it through the Western scientific lens. As stated before, these systems of balance are essential maps that we use to navigate the terrain of physiological and emotional harmony or guide us in the direction of our energetic needs. Now we shift our gaze through the Eastern lens. As we do so, it's important to remember that even though the map looks different and the terminology and language have changed, we are still viewing the same topography: our physical and emotional bodies. We can use these Eastern philosophical views as another tool to understand and ultimately travel toward our desired goals.

There are many different Eastern as well as Western philosophies that can help us navigate.

We will explore three prevalent Eastern yogic philosophies that overlay almost perfectly with the autonomic nervous system and the polyvagal theory:

- **The *nadis*** represent the body's energetic channels in three parts: the *pingala nadi,* which correlates with the sympathetic nervous system; the *ida nadi,* related to the parasympathetic nervous system; and the *sushumna nadi,* which we can compare to a balanced nervous system or the ventral vagal complex. The *nadis* give us a map of our tendencies toward different qualities, characteristics, and attributes. We use this philosophy of the *nadis* with the breath to bring out traits we desire to see in ourselves.

- **The *gunas*** represent how energy is expressed in nature and ourselves. The three *gunas* are like waves that ebb and flow with the tide. Like the *nadis,* the *gunas* correlate with our nervous system and change with the breath. The *gunas* show our energy as it ascends, expands, descends, and contracts through a daily, monthly, and yearly cycle. We can use the *gunas* with our breath to bring us up when we feel low, ground us when we feel scattered, and sustain us in a state of balance and equanimity.

- **The *prana vayus*** represent the movement or flow of energy throughout the body. The five *prana vayus* interact beautifully with all the other systems. Traditionally thought of as how *prana,* or vital life energy, circulates in, out, and through the body, they show us so much more and help create balance where a deficit may be. The *prana vayus* give us insight into our relationship with ourselves and others, our relationship to inner and outer nature, and our relationship to spirituality and our higher self. The map of the *prana vayus* with our breath practice helps guide us to social and interpersonal harmony.

THE *NADIS:* CHANNELS OF ENERGY

Many *pranayama* practices focus on moving energy through the body to create balance, regulate bodily functions, increase strength and stamina, stimulate healing, restore energetic misalignments, guide emotions, and elevate spiritual awareness. There's a common saying in yoga, "Energy goes where the intention flows!" meaning we can move energy through the body by focusing our intention into specific areas.

For example, place both hands in front of your navel as if you're holding a ball. Close your eyes and begin to breathe slowly and deeply. With every inhalation, move your hands slightly apart, and with every exhalation, bring them closer together without allowing your fingers to touch. Imagine a glowing white ball of energy between your hands. As you inhale, visualize the ball growing bigger and pushing your hands farther apart. As you exhale, feel the force of the ball resisting your hands coming together, and as you press your hands toward each other, visualize the ball glowing brighter. Continue with these breath and hand movements for about five minutes while keeping a strong focus and visualization of the energy ball. After five minutes of slow, deep breathing and movement, rest with your hands in the starting position. Keep your eyes closed. Slowly pulse your hands toward and away from each other and feel the energetic resistance between your fingers.

This is a traditional *Qigong* exercise that cultivates the *Qi,* or energy, to be moved and utilized in other practices. If you are still skeptical about the energy practice, you're not alone!

When I first came to yoga, I was somewhat resistant to all the spiritual hippie stuff that goes along with it. I was only there for the physical aspect of the practice; even though I loved breathing exercises and had tried breath retention in the past, when the teachers started talking about energy, *nadis,* or *chakras,* I would tune out. I wanted to see it and feel it, but I was still too closed-minded to allow myself to feel anything subtle like this energy they were talking about. I thought, if you can't cut a body open and see the *chakras* or *nadis* (energy lines), then they weren't really there.

Maybe, to some extent, they are made up, but by shutting them out, I wasn't able to use them as the valuable tool they are. I remember sitting in class doing *nadi shodhana pranayama* (alternate nostril breathing; see pages 132 to 136) and thinking it was silly to close off one nostril because all the air goes to the same place as soon as it passes the septum. I didn't understand that the air I was inhaling was both breath and energy—or that alternate nostril breathing could be a tool to focus the intention from one side to the other to create more balance between my left-side energy *(ida nadi)* and my right-side energy *(pingala nadi).*

I think it's imperative to be skeptical of most things, but it's hard to grow and have new experiences unless you are open to the things you don't know or don't understand. Yoga is a state of connection; everything else is just a tool to help us understand that connection. Whether it's *asana, pranayama, chakras,* or the deity Lord Ganesha, we use the tools that help us when we need them and set aside the ones that aren't useful.

I tend to take a scientific approach to most things. Even with the spiritual side of my practice, I had to find some scientific evidence that would bring the ledge close enough for me to take the leap into the metaphysical, spiritual world.

Spiritual has many connotations depending on whom you talk to, their background, and how they are using the word. We give all words their meaning, and I think it's okay if our meanings vary a bit, although it can be difficult if you are trying to talk about the same thing but have different definitions for what that thing is. So, to give us some common ground, I will define what spirituality means to me, but please feel free to retain your own connection with this word.

For me, *spiritual* describes intangible elements that are beyond my understanding yet are still felt, experienced, and possibly even created through the power of the mind. Spirituality became the impetus to move me past my human limitations to a place of expansion where I could experience a deep and profound connection to nature and all things. As we try to understand the true philosophical questions, like who am I, why am I here, what is my purpose, and what is on the other side of the void, I think it is our spirituality and our connection to the subtle, energetic, and intuitive self that bring us closer to the answers. And for us to sense or move energy, we need to understand our limitations of perception and develop interoception (internal awareness) and intuition.

We have only five senses with which to understand the outside world. Our senses are like little windows that limit how much we can see. And since we can't leave our bodies, we are mostly stuck with this view. Technology has given us the tools to expand our little windows, and now, with these tools, we can see things that were once too far away or too small and even things that we didn't know existed. But we still have many walls we can't see through, so we don't know what's on the other side. Science has already given us a much deeper understanding of the energetic body. It often uses different terminology than the Eastern philosophies, but I believe it is easy to draw the lines that connect the two. And as both science and spirituality grow, the two grow closer together.

How we talk about energy can be confusing. There is the scientific definition that we use to discuss energies like mechanical, electrical, thermal, and chemical. There is also the spiritual definition that refers to *prana* or *Qi.* Some call it the universal force of life, pure love, nature, source, and awareness. So how are they different? Everything we know and see in the physical world was formed with energy, and all living things create and use energy. The beats of my heart are electrical energy; my movement, kinetic energy; the warmth of my skin, thermal energy. My most profound feelings of love come from chemicals like serotonin and dopamine. It might help to separate the types of energy to define and understand them, but it's also helpful to recognize that it's all energy, and however you connect to that understanding of energy is perfect.

Our breath, vitality, and energetic life force are interdependent and interconnected. Therefore, the breath or *prana* is not limited to the lungs. As we inhale, we can direct our *prana* to move anywhere in the body. For example, in a yoga class, the teacher might guide the students to breathe somewhere outside the lungs, like into the belly, the lower back, or even the legs and arms. We use the breath as a vehicle that is guided by an intention to place our awareness in a specific area. While you can send *prana* anywhere in the body just by focusing it there with your mind, *prana* also circulates in a constant state of flow, like water down a river.

Prana travels along pathways called *nadis,* which are channels or conduits, similar to our nervous system. *Nadi* means "nerve" in Sanskrit and comes from the root *nad,* which means "flow, motion, or vibration." The *Hatha Yoga Pradipika,* as well as many other ancient yoga texts, state that there are 72,000 *nadis* throughout the body. (The *Shiva Samhita* describes 350,000, but 72,000 seems to be the more widely adopted philosophy.) Of these *nadis,* the three that are most vital are the *ida, pingala,* and *sushumna.* The *nadis* represent energy channels, but they also represent the archetypes and qualities of the self.

We move energy through the various channels by using our intention. But instead of focusing on "energy" moving through the *nadis,* we focus on a specific quality or multiple qualities that each *nadi* represents. In the beginning, it's easier to focus on one quality at a time. By bringing our attention to certain energetic attributes or emotional qualities, we cultivate those desired aspects within ourselves. For example, if we lack "creativity" and want to inspire it, we can focus on our creative aspect flowing up the *ida nadi,* along the left side of the body since the *ida nadi* represents the innovative and imaginative qualities of the self. Because the *nadis* function as a system of balance, focusing on a quality in the opposing *nadi*, such as the *pingala nadi* if we are concentrating on the *ida nadi*, can help bring more emotional stability overall.

We can do this practice as a meditation or as an intention accompanying any breathing exercise and focusing on the intention while inhaling. We increase the power to cultivate our intention even further when we use a *pranayama* practice that increases the quality of the *nadi*. (See the illustration of *pranayama* effects on pages 154 and 155.)

THE *NADIS*

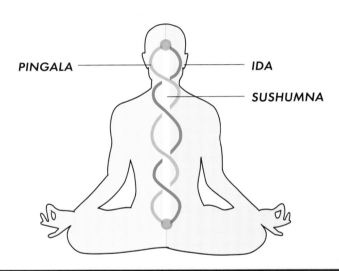

PINGALA ————

———— IDA

———— SUSHUMNA

PINGALA	SUSHUMNA	IDA
"ACTIVE CHANNEL"	"BALANCED CHANNEL"	"PASSIVE CHANNEL"
INHALATION FAST BREATHING	EQUAL BREATHING	EXHALATION SLOW BREATHING
SYMPATHETIC NERVOUS SYSTEM	PARASYMPATHETIC/ VENTRAL VAGAL COMPLEX	PARASYMPATHETIC/ DORSAL VAGAL COMPLEX
YANG ENERGY	YIN/YANG ENERGY	YIN ENERGY
FOCUS	AWARENESS	CREATIVITY
ENERGETIC	EQUANIMITY	INTUITION
OUTGOING	BLISS	RECEPTIVITY

IDA NADI

The *ida nadi,* sometimes referred to as the "passive channel," originates on the left side of the base of the spine at the root *chakra (muladhara chakra)* and spirals upward toward the area behind the eyes, at the third eye *chakra (ajna chakra).* Much like the optic nerve crosses and links the left eye to the right hemisphere of the brain, the *ida* channel crosses at the third eye and is connected to the right brain. Ida represents the lunar or yin subtle energy that is associated with creativity, passivity, receptivity, and intuition. When we are in our *ida* nature, we become more calm and nurturing and tend to be content and relaxed. The *ida nadi* links to the parasympathetic nervous system. When we stimulate the *ida nadi* through *pranayama* practices, we also stimulate the parasympathetic nervous system. Conversely, when we have a more parasympathetic tone, we exhibit more *ida* qualities.

PINGALA NADI

The *pingala nadi,* sometimes referred to as the "active channel," originates on the right side of the base of the spine at the root *chakra* and spirals upward counter to the *ida nadi,* while both intersect and cross along each *chakra* like a double helix up to the area of the third eye *chakra.* Mirroring the *ida* channel, *pingala nadi* connects to the left hemisphere of the brain. *Pingala* represents the solar or yang subtle energy that is associated with logic, power, energy, and assertiveness. When we are in our *pingala* nature, we become more focused, driven, and outgoing and tend to be goal-oriented. When we stimulate our *pingala nadi,* we move more into our sympathetic nervous system. As with the *ida nadi,* this relationship works the other way, too.

SUSHUMNA NADI

Sushumna runs up the center of the spine, starting near the perineum at the root *chakra* and ending at the top of the skull at the junction between the parietal bones and the frontal bone, at the crown *chakra (sahasrara chakra),* and intersects all the *chakras* as it travels upward. *Sushumna* can be called the central energy channel of enlightenment. It is described as a thin, hollow white tube that is usually closed but opens when *ida* and *pingala* are in perfect balance. *Sushumna* then becomes the expression of harmony of the duality of our nature that allows us to realize our higher selves. When we are in our *sushumna* nature, we exhibit wisdom, knowledge, and awareness through a state of bliss and equanimity.

If you've studied the *nadis,* you probably noticed that I didn't refer to *ida* as feminine and *pingala* as masculine, as you would see in almost every yogic text out there. Although some say that masculine and feminine energy are not related to male and female genders, most people associate certain characteristics with a masculine person and certain characteristics with a feminine person. We have very masculine women and men who are very feminine, and vice versa. When I look at the qualities and attributes of *ida* and *pingala,* none of them is unique to a feminine or a masculine person, regardless of sex or gender. As our culture breaks away from gender roles and moves toward equality, I feel that associating feminine energy with being nurturing implies that masculine energy is not nurturing. Likewise, relating masculine energy to being strong and powerful suggests that feminine energy is weak and inferior. These philosophies are outdated and should be rethought to fit our progressive society.

THE *GUNAS:* EXPRESSIONS OF ENERGY

The *gunas* represent the manifestation of consciousness in the form of existence, ranging from the subtlest forms of thought and higher consciousness to the most substantial kinds of physical matter. They are the energetic expression of the essential qualities and attributes of all life. We define each of the three *gunas* by its action or process of movement in the continuous flow of ascending, expanding, descending, and contracting. These actions lay out a guide for us to understand the harmonic flow and turbulent flux that is present in nature and in ourselves. The *gunas* move in cycles that circulate around us, through our outer environment, and within us, through our mind and body—always changing to move toward growth or decay, which results in a struggle for dominance or balance. When we fully understand the effects of the *gunas* and are in a state of conscious awareness, we can change our thoughts and actions to achieve a state of peace and harmony.

As we move to understand the *gunas,* it's important to recognize that they are not some mystical philosophy that was relevant only in ancient India. Instead, they are a significant systematic guide to our physical and emotional attributes, a way to understand the self for the purpose of living a more conscious and healthy life.

I think this description will make a lot more sense once we dive into the attributes of each *guna* and break down this philosophical map.

THE *GUNAS*

SATTVA	*RAJAS*	*TAMAS*
"TO BE"	"TO DO"	"TO HAVE"
BALANCED BREATHING	INHALATION FAST BREATHING	EXHALATION SLOW BREATHING
PARASYMPATHETIC/ VENTRAL VAGAL COMPLEX	SYMPATHETIC NERVOUS SYSTEM	PARASYMPATHETIC/ DORSAL VAGAL COMPLEX
ASCENDING	EXPANDING	DESCENDING AND CONTRACTING
PRESENCE	PASSION	GROUNDING
CONSCIOUSNESS	WORK/PLAY	RELAXATION
COMPASSION	GOAL-ORIENTED	RECOVERY

SATTVA: TO BE

Sattva, which sits at the top of the *guna* hierarchy, is our energetic vibration that is most often expressed as balance and harmony. The best way to think of *sattva* is as the mode "to be." So the qualities arise from a place of tranquility and contentment. There is nowhere to go, nothing to do, and nothing outside of the here and now. This affinity toward presence gives rise to a higher state of consciousness and awareness that leads to joy, love, and compassion. Here we learn that happiness comes from within.

Sattva is always seeking the truth, which is the present moment, and therefore represents ascending movement and growth, specifically spiritual growth and evolution. And it is when we are most balanced that we can reach our highest potential. The *sattva guna* is related to a healthy functional autonomic nervous system. The *sattva guna* works mainly with the ventral vagal complex of the parasympathetic nervous system, which is, as discussed earlier, the state of healthy social engagement. Most autonomic nervous system dysfunctions are a result of chronic stimulation of the sympathetic nervous system, so releasing the stress factors that are causing excessive sympathetic tone and increasing parasympathetic tone will bring our autonomic nervous system into a *sattvic* state.

RAJAS: TO DO

As *sattva* ascends through the cycle of the *gunas,* it naturally moves into the second *guna, rajas. Rajas* is the energy of expansion, always moving outward toward exhaustion. *Rajas* is the mode "to do." We always want to be busy and moving toward something. Our motivation, goals, and accomplishments come from this type of energy. In a healthy flow, *rajas* is essential for daily life; it gets us up and moving. When we balance *rajas* with sattva, we are playful, passionate, sensual, and full of joy. But without *sattva, rajas* moves toward its dark side. This goal-oriented energy becomes obsessed with pleasure-seeking, which can lead to addiction. We become greedy, selfish, and ego-centric. *Rajas* is restless and easily dissatisfied. We are biologically designed to seek pleasure but never be satisfied. Every goal we accomplish comes with a fleeting feeling of satisfaction that is quickly replaced with a need to do more. Our inability to find a lasting resolve is the dilemma of trying to find happiness in our achievements.

Rajas correlates to the sympathetic nervous system. Together, they work to motivate and move us to explore the vast array of beauty this world has to offer. When we remain in *rajas* for too long, the always-doing state chronically stimulates the sympathetic nervous system. We can feel like we are giving a lot of effort but not seeing the results, so we continue to spin our wheels without going anywhere, perpetuating the feeling of not doing enough or being good enough. *Rajas* is associated with fire, and as the fire burns itself out, it descends toward the final *guna, tamas.*

TAMAS: TO HAVE

Tamas is at the bottom of the *guna* cycle, but it shares equal importance with *rajas.* As *rajas* moves into expansion, *tamas* brings it back, first by grounding and then by gathering. It is the descending and contracting movement that polarizes *rajas* and completes the flow. A healthy state of *tamas* is vital to balancing the overactive *rajasic* energy. It acts as our brakes and allows us to practice restraint and self-control. As we slow down, we begin to move into a state of rest and recovery. The descending energy progresses to the bottom of the circle, where it loops back to meet the ascending *sattvic* energy on the upward curve, and this synergy allows us to heal and repair. The mode for *tamas* is "to have." Unlike *rajas,* which is obsessed with getting more, *tamas* wants to hoard everything it has. Having and not wanting more makes us lazy and lethargic. When we remain in *tamas* for too long, we start to develop illness, pain, and other health issues. Tamas is the *guna* of death, which is why it sits at the bottom of the *guna* totem pole.

Tamas correlates with the dorsal vagal complex of the parasympathetic nervous system. As discussed earlier, the dorsal vagal complex regulates the functions of our abdominal organs below the diaphragm, promotes states of deep relaxation, and is responsible for the freeze response. Together, *tamas* and the dorsal vagal complex facilitate stillness, grounding, and tranquility. But when we stay in this state too long, the imbalance leads to apathy, dullness, digestive issues, and over-eating. Tamas then continues to contract, and the emotional dysfunctions of the dorsal vagal complex lead to us feel alienated and depressed.

THE CYCLES OF THE *GUNAS*

The three aspects represented by the *gunas* share a common thread with many Eastern teachings that lead away from consumerism and productivity as primary goals. Instead, the *gunas* emphasize balance and presence. In Western culture, the *rajas* mode "to do" is the prominent topic of many motivational speakers and self-help experts who inspire us to move toward goals and accomplishments as if these achievements will make us happy. Our modern consumer culture aligns with the *tamasic* mode of "to have" that asserts stuff and comfort equal happiness. While both of these modes are necessary and nothing is wrong or evil with either "to do" or "to have," the mode of "to be" is the only one in which we find pure joy and contentment.

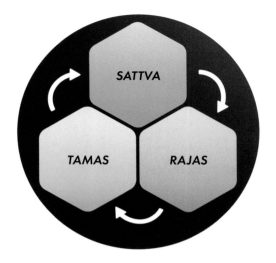

The *gunas* divide the self into three separate aspects:

- **The mental aspect** governs all thinking and logic.

- **The emotional aspect** regulates our mood, affect, and desires.

- **The physical aspect** controls the body.

We can express different *gunas* at the same time through these aspects of the self. For example, the mental aspect can be in *rajas,* the emotional aspect can be in *sattva,* and the physical aspect can be in *tamas.* We might simultaneously experience all three *gunas* as we try to go to sleep. Emotionally, we can feel as though we are in a balanced state of *sattva.* Our bodies can be physically exhausted from a long day and deep in *tamas,* ready for sleep and recovery. Yet we might lie awake for hours, unable to sleep because our minds are busy in *rajas,* thinking about our to-do lists for the next day. Of the *gunas* being expressed, we generally have a dominant *guna,* which depends on which aspect of the self is being emphasized. Each *guna* is in movement, forced by the natural polarity of ascending and descending, expanding and contracting to search for balance. And it is through this movement that the *gunas* form cycles. These cycles are divided into three time frames:

- **Daily,** through a twenty-four-hour period

- **Monthly,** following the twenty-eight-day moon cycle

- **Yearly,** following the seasons

We track the daily cycle from when we wake up until we go to sleep, although the *guna* cycle continues even as we move through REM sleep, light sleep, and deep sleep. The daily cycle is the most prominent of the three and therefore is the easiest to track. During this cycle, the average person remains in each *guna* for approximately two hours before entering the next *guna.* As you become more aware of your *gunas,* you'll be able to control which *guna* you're in longer, especially once you learn how to influence your *gunas* through breathing exercises, which is the easiest and quickest way to change them.

Sattva guna is where we experience the most spiritual growth, awareness, and intelligence, so naturally, we want to be in this *guna* the longest. But because *sattva*'s mode is "to be," this state is incredibly challenging to maintain. The longer we practice presence, the stronger the urge to move and be active becomes; this is especially true in the mental aspect of self, which gravitates toward *rajas* faster than the emotional and physical aspects. *Sattva* ascends until we reach the energetic height of our conscious limit; it then flows into *rajas* where *rajas* expands outward. People with an abundance of energy, excitement, and joy tend to be able to maintain *rajas* energy for long periods. Once our energy is exhausted, *rajas* falls toward *tamas* to rest and recovery. If we push too hard and too long in *rajas,* then the fall to *tamas* lands with a big crash, from which it can take a long time to recover. Over-exertion extends the *rajas* and *tamas* cycles and shortens our ability to maintain a *sattvic* state.

Tamas gathers energy to recharge the batteries and make repairs. People who can sit still in meditation or deep relaxation for a long time are able to maintain an extended healthy state of *tamas.* Once we restore our energy and feel rejuvenated, we move back into *sattva,* and the cycle starts over. But if rest and recovery become laziness and lethargy, then it generally takes a strong push from *rajas* to pull us out, and we completely skip the *sattvic* state. Many people spend the majority of their daily cycle in the inactivity that is encompassed by the *tamasic* state. You can also bounce back and forth between being in *rajas* and *tamas* without ever experiencing *sattva.* This happens when we become so focused on doing and having that we forget about being and enjoying.

Ideally, we learn how to balance *rajas* and *tamas* as well as use these energies in positive ways that bring benefits to our lives and our needs. Then we can increase our ability to maintain a *sattvic* state and remain in the true happiness that comes from within.

To use the *gunas* as a tool to understand your energetic cycle and affect this cycle to improve your life, I think it's helpful to start by noticing which *guna* you are in when you wake up. If you wake up feeling rested and balanced, then you're in the *sattva guna.* If you wake up with a ton of energy, ready to take on the day, then you're in *rajas.* If you wake up and you hit snooze five times, force yourself out of bed, and can't talk to anyone until you've had your coffee, you're in *tamas.*

I prefer to wake up in *sattva* because I do my meditation first thing in the morning and then a *pranayama* practice that brings me into *rajas* so I feel energized for my morning yoga practice and the activities of the day. I also try to go to sleep in a *sattva/tamas* state. If you are going to sleep in *tamas,* you want to guide yourself into this *guna* by doing breathing exercises and relaxation techniques. It's generally not good to go to sleep feeling *tamasic* because you have exhausted all your *rajasic* energy. Usually, if you go to sleep in *tamas* because you're exhausted, you'll also wake up in *tamas* feeling exhausted. *Rajas* is the worst energy to try to fall asleep in, especially when the mental aspect is in *rajas* but the physical body is in *tamas.* This is a prevalent stress state for people: the body is exhausted but the mind won't stop spinning.

The daily cycle is influenced by the underlying pull of the monthly and yearly cycles, much like the waves and tides of the ocean will alter the course of a boat but not necessarily change its direction. We feel a gradual change from one *guna* to another, with each *guna* lasting seven to fourteen days, but one *guna* can also span an entire month. The transitions of the *gunas* through the monthly cycle match the physical and emotional changes that women go through during their menstrual cycle, with *tamas* being the most dominant during their period. Men also feel the effects of the *gunas* changing in the monthly cycle as the moon affects all of us, but in general, women are affected more by the monthly cycle and men are affected more by the yearly cycle.

The yearly cycle also has a general pull on how we experience the daily *guna* cycle. This influence on the *gunas* correlates with the change of the seasons and the lengths of the days. Longer, warmer days give us more *rajasic* energy, and shorter, cooler days give us more *tamasic* energy. The yearly cycle has a more substantial effect in places where there are more dramatic changes in seasons and is less apparent in areas where the climate is more temperate.

THE *PRANA VAYUS:*
A SYSTEM OF RELATIONSHIPS

The *prana vayus* are both a system and a map of energy flow through the body. When the system is in balance, it works to regulate all bodily functions, such as breathing, circulation, and digestion, and is closely related to the autonomic nervous system. You could even say that the *prana vayus* were the ancient yogis' interpretation of how the sympathetic and parasympathetic nervous systems govern the body, as the two theories are almost identical.

Like the autonomic nervous system, the *vayus* are interconnected with our emotions. The *vayus,* or internal winds, give us a way to view and understand how imbalances and blockages manifest as physical maladies and emotional dysfunction. They provide insight on how to restore and maintain harmony within ourselves, in our relationships with others, and with our higher self. Although they are taught in many ways, with the details differing slightly (or sometimes quite a bit among the various lineages), most teachings of the *prana vayus* arrive at the same place.

There are five *vayus* that correlate to *prana* (energy) entering, circulating, and leaving the body. Like all energies, *prana* is healthiest when it is flowing.

THE *PRANA VAYUS*

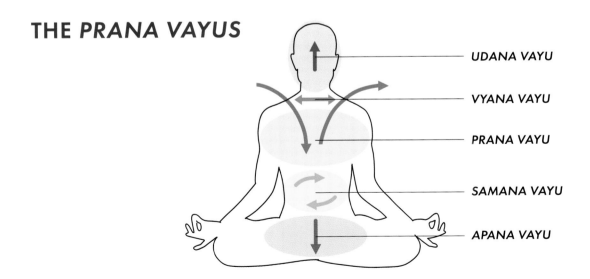

UDANA VAYU

VYANA VAYU

PRANA VAYU

SAMANA VAYU

APANA VAYU

UDANA VAYU	VYANA VAYU	PRANA VAYU	SAMANA VAYU	APANA VAYU
UPWARD FLOW OF ENERGY	EXPANDING FLOW OF ENERGY	INWARD/OUTWARD FLOW OF ENERGY	CONTRACTING FLOW OF ENERGY	DOWNWARD FLOW OF ENERGY
BALANCED BY *APANA VAYU*	BALANCED BY *SAMANA VAYU*	SELF-BALANCING	BALANCED BY *VYANA VAYU*	BALANCED BY *UDANA VAYU*
INHALATION	INHALATION	INHALATION/ EXHALATION	EXHALATION	EXHALATION
SYMPATHETIC NERVOUS SYSTEM	SYMPATHETIC NERVOUS SYSTEM	PARASYMPATHETIC/ VENTRAL VAGAL COMPLEX	PARASYMPATHETIC/ DORSAL VAGAL COMPLEX	PARASYMPATHETIC/ DORSAL VAGAL COMPLEX
CONSCIOUSNESS	CREATIVITY	EQUANIMITY	WELL-BEING	GROUNDING
HIGHER SELF AND SPIRITUALITY	POSITIVE EMOTIONS	RELATIONSHIP OF INNER AND OUTER NATURE	RELATIONSHIP TO SELF	RELEASE AND NON-ATTACHMENT
COMMUNICATION	RELATIONSHIPS	CONNECTION	BALANCE	INTIMACY

If you leave your cell phone for a week without using or charging it, it will go dead. If you use it nonstop, it will die even quicker. If you overload the battery, the phone might catch fire. But when your charging and usage are balanced, your phone functions as intended. Energy needs a similar kind of input and output to flow and maintain balance. If a surplus exists in one area, a deficit likely resides in the other. The *vayus* help us understand the flow and how to adjust for imbalances.

As we visualize the energetic flow of each *vayu,* we begin to understand how the emotional qualities link to the direction of movement as well as the relationship with ourselves or others.

PRANA VAYU

Prana vayu is the first of the energetic winds and arguably the most important, which could be why it shares its name with the collective of the *vayus.* While the other four *vayus* form a system of balancing themselves as well as working to create balance with another contrasting *vayu, prana vayu* is unique in that it is the only one that balances itself with itself.

Prana vayu represents the inward and outward flow of energy as it enters and leaves the body. Another way to look at it is that *prana vayu* is the inhalation and the exhalation. It is the exchange of outer *prana* entering the body and inner *prana* leaving the body. It represents the relationship between our outer nature and our inner nature, as this continuous exchange creates a union between the two that brings us closer to source nature, which is the whole and the belief that we are not separate.

When *prana vayu* is out of balance, we can feel out of place and not understand our purpose in this life. Our meaning of life comes from how we define our connection to our role within the whole. We often feel like something is missing, so we seek to fill the hole with things that will never make us feel more whole. Balancing *prana vayu* brings us back to the truth that we are whole to begin with, and you cannot add anything or take anything away to make you more you. We return to being a part of the whole rather than apart from the whole.

To balance *prana vayu,* inhale through your nose without creating any restriction. As you fill your chest, visualize the purest air flowing from nature into your lungs. Feel the connection to the breath as you hold it in for a few moments. Slowly exhale as you feel your place in and connection to the world. Continue this breathing practice as a meditation where you focus on your inner and outer nature being the same.

After *prana* enters the body via *prana vayu* and before exiting, also by way of *prana vayu,* it is circulated throughout the body via the other four *vayus,* which are *apana vayu, udana vayu, vyana vayu,* and *samana vayu.*

APANA VAYU

Apana vayu is the descending flow of energy, and it primarily has to do with the elimination of waste, negative emotions, and intimacy. Dysfunctions of *apana vayu* come from not wanting to release the things that are no longer serving us or from unwanted changes in things that bring us happiness. Consequently, resisting these changes assists in forming our attachments. Attachment is very different from connection, even though they sound like synonyms. Connection is fluid; when we understand our interconnectedness to the whole, we change, morph, and evolve continuously as everything else also continually changes. Therefore, when we remain in flux and flow, we can experience true freedom. Attachment, however, arises from our desire for things to stay the same and our resistance to change. Unfortunately, everything is continuously changing, and our attachments only lead to separation, which causes suffering, stress, and anxiety.

Apana vayu is most closely associated with the autonomic nervous system and the vagus nerve, especially when in healthy function. A blockage with *apana vayu* can lead to a chronically stimulated sympathetic nervous system. We see this manifest in the body as problems with constipation, impotence, and menstrual complications. Mentally, blockages show up as our inability to let go of emotional baggage, holding on to or continuously revisiting past traumas, and lack of spiritual growth. When *apana vayu* is in healthy flow, digestion and elimination are also in healthy flow.

Emotionally, we can let go of the negative aspects of the past and move forward toward spiritual growth. We feel less stress and anxiety and readily accept change. *Apana vayu* also gives us our sense of being grounded and connected to the earth and our physical form.

To balance *apana vayu,* inhale slowly and deeply for a count of five to ten seconds. Allow a slight natural pause before exhaling. Exhale for double the length of the inhalation. As you exhale, think about letting go of all contractions in the body and visualize space and expansion in your chest and belly. Continue the practice until you feel yourself in a state of calm and deep relaxation. It is best to do this practice while lying on your back.

UDANA VAYU

Udana vayu is the upward spiraling flow of energy and translates as "the air that flies up." *Udana vayu* is our relationship to source, consciousness, and our higher self. It is connected to our five senses, through which we form our perception of the world. *Udana vayu* is the energy of expression and communication. It allows us to share our thoughts, feelings, and emotions in an open and honest way. When it's balanced, it manifests as joy and enthusiasm for life and often is expressed through singing, chanting, and laughter. Blockages in *udana vayu* can make it challenging to communicate honestly and openly with others. We can feel shut-in or stuck in place. We feel like no one listens to us, and when they do, they misinterpret our words. Physically, blockages in *udana vayu* can create problems with hearing and swallowing and often lead to poor diets that are high in salt, sugar, and fat.

To balance or unblock *udana vayu,* take a full inhalation slowly through your nose. As you inhale, visualize the breath coming up through the soles of your feet, up your legs, pelvis, and spine until it reaches the level of the throat where your vocal cords are. Place your tongue against the soft palate in the roof of your mouth; sing the sound "om" with your mouth closed as you slowly exhale out the nose. Focus on the feeling of love and joy in your heart and visualize a bright white light between your eyes. Hold your breath for several seconds at the bottom of the exhalation until you feel the need to inhale again. Repeat this practice until you feel joy, ease, and clarity.

Udana vayu and *apana vayu* share a close relationship in balancing each other. *Apana vayu* acts as the anchor to prevent *udana vayu* from flying away, and *udana vayu* keeps *apana vayu* from sinking too deep into itself. When there is a surplus in *udana* and a deficit in *apana,* we tend to live with our head in the clouds with no basis in reality. Too much *apana vayu* and not enough *udana vayu,* and we become set in our ways and resistant to any kind of growth and change.

VYANA VAYU

Vyana vayu distributes the current of energy throughout the body and into the extremities as it flows through the 72,000 *nadis* (refer to pages 65 to 70). *Vyana vayu* is associated with the somatic nervous system, which controls our muscles, and the parts of the autonomic nervous system that control breathing, circulation, and heart functions. It links to all the nerves and blood vessels that run through the body and helps maintain and regulate the healthy functions of muscles and joints. *Vyana vayu* manifests as creativity, talent, and positive emotions. It is associated with our outward flow of energy that is felt and received by others. This positive flow of love and energy enables us to form stable and healthy relationships with others. Blockages in *vyana vayu* can lead to cardiac problems, high blood pressure, and respiratory problems, as well as muscle fatigue, weakness, and joint pain. Emotionally, they make us feel uninspired, secluded, separate, and alone.

To balance *vyana vayu,* bring your awareness to your heart space. Imagine your heart is breathing instead of your lungs. With every inhalation, draw pure love into the center of your heart. As you exhale, radiate loving energy through every part of the body, extending outward past your skin and to all the people you care for and love. Allow your breath to be soft and relaxed throughout the practice as you focus on the powerful intention of love.

SAMANA VAYU

Samana vayu brings energy back to the center of the body and functions to regulate and maintain balance of the energetic flow of the other *vayus,* especially between *prana vayu* and *apana vayu.* Energetically, *samana vayu* exists near the solar plexus. *Samana* means "the same" or "equal." It gives us a sense of equilibrium and balance as well as inner well-being. It governs the stomach, liver, spleen, and pancreas and is responsible for the digestion and absorption of nutrients. Emotionally, it has to do with self-identity, willpower, and self-love. When *samana vayu* is blocked, we can feel lazy and lethargic. It can lead to malnutrition, slow metabolism, eating disorders, and obesity. These dysfunctions often arise from low self-esteem, low self-worth, and a lack of self-love. We feel hopeless, afraid, unmotivated, and powerless to change our situation, which leads us deeper into a state of depression.

Keeping *samana vayu* free and open is important because dysfunction here sends the rest of the *vayus* into a downward spiral. To unblock and reconnect *samana vayu,* we practice four-part equal breathing. With a slow inhalation, completely fill the lungs. Focus on examining the breath in all directions, deep into the pelvis, low back, belly, upper back, chest, and collarbones. Count the time it takes to take a full, slow, deep breath. Hold your breath for the same amount of time as the inhalation and imagine the *prana* being pushed throughout your entire body. Exhale fully, equal to the length of the in-breath. Hold your breath at the bottom of the exhalation for the same count and visualize the *prana* returning inward, toward the center of your solar plexus. Do a few rounds until you feel comfortable with the breath count and can match the lengths of each part of the breath without having to focus on counting. Repeat the mantra, "I am love! I love that I am love!"

As well as being a governing energy for the *vayus, samana vayu* holds a deep relationship to the balance of *vyana vayu. Samana vayu* is primarily about our relationship with ourselves, whereas *vyana vayu* has to do with our relationships with others. When we are able to accept and love ourselves fully, we are also able to accept and love others fully. Imbalances between these two vayus can lead to a continual search for validation, love, and acceptance from others because of our inability to love ourselves. Or it can result in self-centered narcissism, where we have a total disregard for others' well-being.

The *prana vayus* act as a complete system of energetic, physical, and emotional balance. If one *vayu* is blocked, depleted, or overactive, it can have a cascading effect that knocks the other *vayus* out of whack. The *prana vayus* also show us how interconnected our energetic/emotional body and our physical body are. To live a happy and free life, we have to focus our efforts on the whole system, not just one aspect. I see the *vayus* as placing us in the chain of connection between our inner and outer natures, our grounded and our spiritual selves, and the interdependent relationship between you and me. The health of our physical body and nervous system directly impacts our moods, emotions, and relationships. Studies have shown that just thinking positive thoughts can lower stress, decrease sympathetic activity, increase parasympathetic activity, and restore autonomic function, which has a profoundly positive effect on our cardiorespiratory system, digestive system, and emotional state.[3]

PUTTING THE SYSTEMS TOGETHER

The autonomic nervous system is the body's physical expression of energy. The *nadis, gunas,* and *vayus* are emotional expressions of the same energetic body. All four systems are interconnected and reference the same thing: how we move into a place of balance and harmony and what happens when our energy is blocked, out of alignment, or in dysfunction. Each system shows us a slightly different map of the physical and emotional body and what happens when we put too much energy into one area or create a deficit in another. And while the practices in this book have a direct and profound effect on restoring, rejuvenating, and balancing our physical and energetic bodies, they work far better when we also address the causes of other imbalances in our lives. I hope the breath can bring you to a deeper state of awareness and be a powerful tool to create positive changes in your life.

The union of the Eastern and Western systems of energy is reflected in the effects of the breathing practice. Just as the breath has a direct correlation to the autonomic nervous system, it has the same connection to the *nadis* and the *gunas.* Although the systems use different approaches to map out behaviors of balance and dysfunction, when we come from an energetic and breath approach, we see that they are stimulated in the same way. The inhalation increases energy while the exhalation decreases energy, and balancing the inhalation and exhalation balances energy. When we have a surplus or deficit, we look to the opposite side of the scale to see where we can find balance either by adding or taking away.

The autonomic nervous system, when understood through the polyvagal theory, has three branches or divisions:

- **The sympathetic nervous system** is related to increasing energy and linked to the inhalation.

- **The dorsal vagal complex** of the parasympathetic nervous system is connected to decreasing energy and is linked to the exhalation.

- **The ventral vagal complex** of the parasympathetic nervous system is related to balance and is associated with a balance between the inhalation and the exhalation and breath retention.

The three central *nadis* follow the same division of energetic flow:

- *Pingala* is the dynamic channel. It links to many of the qualities of the sympathetic nervous system and is excited through the inhalation.

- *Ida* is the calming, more restorative channel. It is linked to the dorsal vagal complex and is stimulated by the exhalation and retention after the exhalation.

- *Sushumna* represents balance and equanimity and correlates to the ventral vagal complex. Just like the ventral branch, balancing the breath and breath retention guide us deeper into this state.

When we view the characteristics of the *gunas,* again, we see similar (though slightly different) expressions of energy:

- **Sattva** represents upward energy in the relationship to spiritual growth. Even though the energy is flowing upward, its mode of "to be" is in relation to balance, and the characteristics of *sattva* are balance and harmony. *Sattva* energetically aligns with the harmonious state of the *sushumna nadi* and the ventral vagal complex.

- The expanding energy of **rajas** increases toward a state of exhaustion. It is stimulated by the inhalation, sharing many of the same energetic qualities as the *pingala nadi* and the sympathetic nervous system.

- **Tamas** closely mirrors the dorsal vagal complex and shares the more passive qualities with the *ida nadi,* also following the exhalation.

The *prana vayus* respond to the breath and movement of energy slightly differently from the previous three systems, although they share many similarities:

- **Prana vayu** is most similar to the ventral vagal complex and the energy systems that orientate around balance since *prana vayu* is the movement from out to in and in to out, it is the inhalation and the exhalation.

- **Apana vayu** moves with the downward flow of energy and the exhalation. We see how it links to the dorsal vagal complex, the *tamas guna,* and the *ida nadi.*

- **Udana vayu** is the upward flow of energy and flows with the inhalation.

- **Vyana vayu** also follows the inhalation. *Vyana* expands from the center and moves outward and shares the energetic movement with *rajas.*

- **Samana vayu** gathers the energy back to the center and moves with the exhale in the same way that *tamas* moves to gather and contract.

A former anatomy professor of mine explained that the difference between anatomy and physiology is like knowing how to read a map and knowing how to use one. We need to know how to do both. We need to know how to read the map to navigate toward our destination. We also need to understand where we are going, why we want to get there, and the vehicles available to take us there. In other words, if we know the map but not its real-world application, then the map is useless. With our baseline knowledge of the physiology of breathing and the systems of balance, we can start exploring the different breathing techniques that will carry us to our goals of improved health, cognitive function, and emotional well-being.

SYSTEMS OF BALANCE

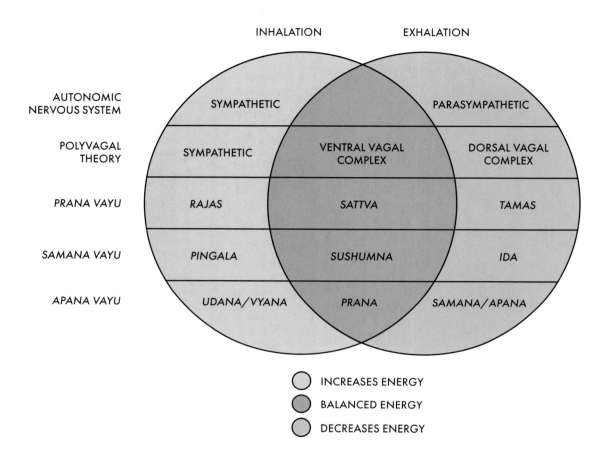

INHALATION   EXHALATION

	INHALATION		EXHALATION
AUTONOMIC NERVOUS SYSTEM	SYMPATHETIC		PARASYMPATHETIC
POLYVAGAL THEORY	SYMPATHETIC	VENTRAL VAGAL COMPLEX	DORSAL VAGAL COMPLEX
PRANA VAYU	RAJAS	SATTVA	TAMAS
SAMANA VAYU	PINGALA	SUSHUMNA	IDA
APANA VAYU	UDANA/VYANA	PRANA	SAMANA/APANA

○ INCREASES ENERGY

● BALANCED ENERGY

◐ DECREASES ENERGY

NOTES

[1]Stephen W. Porges, "The polyvagal theory: new insights into adaptive reactions of the autonomic nervous system," *Cleveland Clinic Journal of Medicine* 76, Suppl 2 (2009): S86–90, doi:10.3949/ccjm.76.s2.17.

[2]Patrick R. Steffen, Tara Austin, Andrea DeBarros, and Tracy Brown, "The impact of resonance frequency breathing on measures of heart rate variability, blood pressure, and mood," *Frontiers in Public Health* 5 (2017): 222, doi:10.3389/fpubh.2017.00222.

[3]Willem J. Kop, Stephen J. Synowski, Miranda E. Newell, Louis A. Schmidt, Shari R. Waldstein, and Nathan A. Fox, "Autonomic nervous system reactivity to positive and negative mood induction: the role of acute psychological responses and frontal electrocortical activity," *Biological Psychology* 86, no. 3 (2011): 230–8, doi:10.1016/j.biopsycho.2010.12.003.

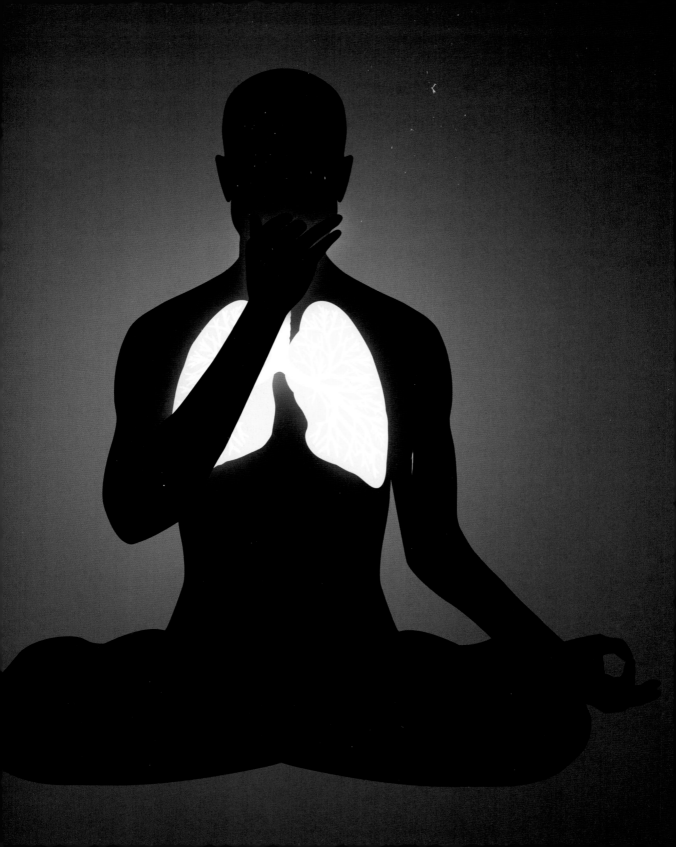

[SECTION 3]
PRANAYAMA: THE YOGIC PRACTICE OF BREATHING

Pranayama is the ancient yogic practice of breath control. The Sanskrit word combines *prana,* meaning "life-force, the breath of life, or vitality," and *ayama,* which means "to control, lengthen, restrain, or extend." Essentially, *pranayama* is the practice of extending, controlling, or expanding the breath to increase our energy, health, and vitality through a series of breathing practices that affect both the physical body and the energetic body.

YOGA: THE PHILOSOPHY OF CONNECTION

Before we dive deeper into *pranayama,* it is helpful to have a brief understanding of how yoga philosophy relates to the breathing practices. One of the most fundamental philosophies of yoga is connection, meaning that the mind, breath, physical body, and energetic body are not separate. More than seeing the self as being connected to itself, yoga views all things in the universe as being interdependent and interconnected. Essentially, all life, nature, animate and inanimate objects, including our thoughts and emotions, affect everything else because of the deep connection that everything shares.

Yoga essentially means "whole." It describes a state of being that recognizes everything as connected. The reason I use the word *whole* and not *yoke* or *join,* which is the more traditional English translation, is that *yoke* and *join* imply two are coming together to form one—as in, we start out separate and then join together to become one. But, much like an embryo begins as a single fertilized cell and multiplies into many individual cells that come together to form one human, the many are what make the one. Another way to say it is that we were not constructed from many parts to make a whole; we were whole to begin with.

Yoga philosophy refers to the world as being under the veil of Maya. *Maya* means "unreality," "fraud," or "deceitful trick"; "illusion" is an easier and maybe a nicer way to say it. For a long time, I thought illusion meant that everything I saw and experienced wasn't real. I would think, how can all this be fake when it feels so real? But illusion doesn't mean that what we see and experience is not real; it just means that reality is not as it appears to us. For example, a good magician performing a trick can fool us into believing that what we're seeing is real. The trick is real, but what we think we are witnessing is different from what is actually happening.

Yoga teaches us that reality, as we see it, is like a giant magic trick—a trick so good that the entire world goes on living and believing that what they see is as it is. This trick is that we are separate. The world appears to be made up of billions of separate entities, but yoga says that it is not. We see it as separate because we view the world through the lens of self, the individual, a part of the bigger whole. It is impossible to see anything not as the self, or outside of the ego. We are all having a subjective experience, and even if we experience some things objectively, meaning that we are not imprinting our past experiences, preferences, or judgments upon reality as it happens outside of us, those experiences are still perceived as we are, just with the understanding that the objective reality is not as we are. To have a truly objective experience is impossible because experience in itself is subjective.

The self creates the illusion of one, and as soon as you identify as one, you have to acknowledge that there are two; this is where the idea of separation comes from. We identify as the self, as a separate entity from other beings, and we create a separation between the self and all other things. The idea of "one" or the concept of "many" comes from our perspective. We can see ourselves as a whole complete human or as a collection of individual cells and microorganisms, as a singularity, or many things making one thing. Here's a fun way to see it: the human body comprises approximately 37 trillion cells.[1] Each cell has a cell wall separating it from the other cells, a nucleus that acts as its brain, and various other organelles that help it perform its function. Each cell is a part of something bigger; even though it works as a separate entity, performing functions ultimately and altruistically, it performs these functions in order for us to live, move, breathe, eat, and reproduce.

On top of the 37 trillion cells that comprise us, it is estimated that we house over 100 trillion bacteria cells[2] that are not us. In fact, our bodies contain more "not us" than "us," yet we don't tend to see ourselves as a collection of separate cells and microorganisms. Compare the trillions of things that make us to the 7.8 billion people living on this planet, whom we see as separate from us. But because we are the ones perceiving, or having the subjective experience, we can only see ourselves as separate. The ultimate path of yoga is to move past the witness of the self to realize we are more than the self; we are the whole.

I don't know if it is possible to transcend the ego to the place where we lose identity of the self entirely and become one with the source, but I know that if we are able to transcend the self, the self will not be able to realize it. There must be an "I" or "ego" to have the experience of realization. If we transcend the self, the one experiencing, then the one having the experience no longer exists. It's more important to understand that we are all whole— not one whole, just whole, interconnected, and interdependent with all of the universe. When we realize this, the individual choices we make will come from the understanding of how everything is affected by our actions. It also helps to understand that *separate* and *different* are not the same thing. We can both be different and connected. To be separate is to be disconnected. To be different only implies uniqueness. My thumb is different from my other fingers and still connected to my hand, but if I cut off my thumb, it becomes separate from my hand.

I explain this yogic nondualism concept of connection because it relates to the practice of *pranayama* in that it helps us understand the much easier concept of the inseparable union between the energetic body and the physical body. As we begin to understand the body better, we can see how the state of our physical body affects how we feel and how the state of our emotional body directly relates to our physical health. An example of this is how stress—a word we often use to describe being unhappy—leads to a weakened immune system, faster aging, and fatigue and can even cause cancer.

The breath is the great link that ties the emotions and the physical body together. Often we can't do much to change our feelings, but we can quickly and easily change the way we breathe, which leads to profound effects, as I will discuss later. The practices in this book affect both the physical and the energetic self, and to fully move toward our intentions through the various exercises, we must focus equally on them both. As we move deeper into the practice of *pranayama,* we begin to manifest the profound, far-reaching effects that breathing can have in our lives. Slightly changing the breath can affect our mood, attitude, clarity of thought, and well-being. Ultimately, all the practices in this book, regardless of the intention, will lead us to a better place of understanding the self.

Pranayama is often linked with meditation, perhaps because many mediation practices have us follow the breath or the sensation of the breath as the object of meditation. Where the breath goes, the mind tends to follow:

- When we are **upset,** we often start to breathe fast and heavy.

- When we are **sad,** we might sigh deeply.

- When we **panic** or are **frightened,** our breath might become short and choppy.

- When we are **calm,** the breath is slow and steady.

While *pranayama* is about controlling the breath, meditation is not about controlling the mind; it is about understanding the tendencies of the mind. It would be nice to think that we are in control of our minds, but if you've ever really tried to control your thoughts, stop your thoughts, or change how you feel, you quickly realize that the mind truly has a mind of its own. The mind is like a dog; a well-trained dog makes you believe that you are in control. If you say sit, it sits. If you say stay, it stays—but as soon as another dog or cat runs by, the dog goes after it! Of course, the better trained the dog is, the more obedient it is, and maybe it won't run after everything that it instinctually wants to chase.

When we see children and even many adults, we know how the smallest outside stimulus can quickly turn their world upside down. One aggressively chosen finger shown to someone else can quickly change their relaxed demeanor into a fit of rage. Meditation helps train the mind to be less reactive and more active. The better we train the mind, the more "control" we have over it. And for the things that are outside our ability to avoid reacting to, we have the breath to bring us back.

> " WHEN THE **BREATH IS UNSTEADY**, THE **MIND IS UNSTEADY**. WHEN THE **BREATH IS STEADY**, THE **MIND IS STEADY**, AND THE **YOGI BECOMES STEADY**. THEREFORE, ONE SHOULD **RESTRAIN THE BREATH**.
>
> —Svatmarama, the *Hatha Yoga Pradipika* (translated)[3] "

BRINGING THE POWER OF INTENTION TO THE BREATH

Pranayama is a practice of conscious breathing whereby we change the depth, rate, rhythm, and quality of each breath to move toward an intention. While each *pranayama* practice might have a general purpose, these motives can be vague and misleading. It's really the intention that we place upon the practice that moves us toward our desired results. As explained in Section 1, every breath we take creates a physiological response, from cellular respiration to a change in blood pH. The same breath also generates an energetic response from the autonomic nervous system and our emotional body, which is the physical perception of chemicals and hormones, expressed as emotions; this is the focus of Section 2. When we realize that everything we know and experience is experienced emotionally and that our emotions are just a physiological response to our actions and environment, we are able to take control of the energy that forms us and shape it to our needs, desires, and passions. Clear intentions give us clear results. If you set out on a path and you don't know where it leads, it can take you anywhere, which is not necessarily a bad thing. But when you know where you want to go, you have to find and follow the path that is going to take you there.

Some *pranayama* exercises are often combined with *mudras,* which are hand gestures that focus energy and direct the intention. Yoga has several hundred *mudras,* each with a unique purpose and intention. While the subtleties of the *mudras* with their claims of creating profound effects can seem foreign and strange, they are not far from what we already know and practice. Western culture has its own *mudras.* Placing the palms together in front of the heart is a *mudra* that shows gratitude and humility. When we make this gesture toward someone, they feel our intention. The same goes if we raise a middle finger; although the intention is very different, the negative energy is strongly felt. The middle finger doesn't have any power on its own, but the energy and intention we give it does. And by simply lifting the index finger, the negative energy is transformed to convey peace. A *mudra* is a tool that can be used to help the mind direct energy according our intention. Without the intention, *mudras* are just hand signals. But with intention, they can harness the power of the mind. So, when we practice a *pranayama* exercise that involves using a *mudra,* we don't place the focus on the *mudra;* instead, we use the *mudra* as a tool to direct our focus.

I'll include more information about various *mudras* with the specific breath practices that employ them, later in this section.

THE COMPONENTS OF THE BREATH

Earlier in the book, we touched on the four parts of the breath cycle—the inhalation, inner retention, exhalation, and outer retention—in order to discuss how they affect the energies of the body. Here, we are going to expand upon this concept and add in the Sanskrit term for each part. Learning and understanding these terms can be valuable, as Sanskrit gives us insight into the subtler qualities that can be associated with breathing. I also find it much easier to use Sanskrit words to instruct the different types of breath retention because Sanskrit has words that directly describe these components, whereas English does not.

PURAKA—INHALATION

Puraka is the Sanskrit word for the inhalation. When translated literally, *puraka* means "satisfying," "filling," or "fulfilling." You often hear or see it as *puraka pranayama,* which gives the intention of the inhalation; to breathe is not just about filling up our lungs, but it's a gratifying act that brings enjoyment. When we inhale with this sentiment, we can immediately feel a positive change in mood, and the effects ripple through our energetic body. *Puraka* can also refer to the receiving and gathering of *prana* and spiritual knowledge; as previously discussed, the breath is more than just the air we breathe.

RECHAKA—EXHALATION

Rechaka or *recaka* (in Sanskrit, *c* is always pronounced "ch") means "to release the breath or exhale." It evokes an emptying, emitting, or purging. *Rechaka* is the basis of many philosophies and provides the energetic movement to support many of these ideas. Yoga teaches us that having attachments always leads to suffering. To be attached to something or someone means that we are looking for happiness in that thing or person staying the same. Because change is the universal truth, anything we are attached to will eventually change, and that change will bring about separation, which is the root of suffering. Instead, we let go of the things we were never able to hold on to in the first place. By letting go, we are able to see the connection that is fluid with change, just as the ocean allows the waves to move freely. The waves change, but their connection to the ocean remains.

A way to understand the difference between attachment and connection is to remember someone you've lost. When you lose someone you love, you immediately feel the pain that is caused by separation. The pain associated with the attachment fades over time. After the pain is gone, all that is left is the love and connection, which never fades. Buddhism emphasizes emptiness, or *sunyata,* as an essential part of liberation and enlightenment. Only through emptiness can we realize spaciousness and begin to see the underlying connection that exists beyond our attachments. *Rechaka* has a beautiful way of showing us how to release the things that aren't serving us. We symbolically and energetically exhale to free ourselves of those things we no longer want to hold on to.

Puraka and *rechaka* interact in a beautiful dance where filling needs emptying and emptying needs filling. This simple interaction teaches us some of the most valuable lessons of the Buddha on freeing ourselves from suffering. We don't try to get rid of the things we have but don't want, and we don't try to obtain the things we want but don't have. The inhalation will never last, and we can never truly get rid of the exhalation. Instead, we see things as they are, existing in the continuously changing, interconnected reality.

KUMBHAKA—RETENTION

Kumbhaka translates as "pot" or "container," and it refers to any practice where we hold the breath and retain the *prana*. *Kumbhaka* is considered the most important of the *pranayama* practices and a way to live longer.

The ancient yogis developed many techniques and philosophies from being in deep communion with nature. The *asana,* or postural practice of yoga, has many poses named after animals that yogis observed in nature. They noticed the animals that breathed fast died much faster than the slow-breathing animals. The slower an animal breathed, the longer its life span was. For example, the longest-living mammal on record, the bonehead whale, has an average life span of 200 years. The bonehead whale breathes only once or twice per minute while resting at the surface and four to six times per minute before preparing for a dive, and then it can hold its breath for up to an hour. In contrast, a mouse breathes up to 230 times per minute and lives only one to three years. The giant tortoise, the longest-living land animal breathing four to six times per minute, is referenced in the Vedas and the Bhagavad Gita.

Krishna, the Hindu god in the Bhagavad Gita, states that by practicing *kumbhaka,* yogis could increase their life span by many years. The ancient yogis believed that we are limited to a certain number of breaths in a lifetime, and if we learn how to breathe slower, we can live longer. As we develop an understanding of the physiology of breathing and the positive effects that come from building up and retaining carbon dioxide, it's easy to see the truth in what the yogis predicted thousands of years ago. Breathing slower and holding our breath improves our health and our chances of living a long, healthy life.

The three major types of *kumbhaka* are *antara kumbhaka, bahya kumbhaka,* and *kevala kumbhaka.*

ANTARA KUMBHAKA—INNER RETENTION

Antara kumbhaka, which means "full container," is the breath retention after inhalation, when our lungs are completely full, or at our vital capacity. (Retaining the breath between the full point and the empty point is referred to as just *kumbhaka.*) *Antara kumbhaka* is the easiest of the breath retentions because we are holding the most air for cellular respiration.

There are two ways to retain the breath on the inhalation. The first is to constrict the glottis and close the vocal cords, which creates a seal and doesn't allow air to escape. We can then relax our diaphragm and the accessory muscles of inhalation. This technique makes it easier to hold the breath for longer periods because it requires less effort. When we release the hold, we hear a little aspirated "ahh" sound.

The second and probably less familiar way is to hold *antara kumbhaka* while leaving the trachea open, without constricting the glottis. This retention is done by using the diaphragm and accessory muscles to expand the chest and then hold the expansion with muscle control. This technique is great for strengthening the diaphragm and the accessory muscles. However, it takes more effort, and holding the breath is much harder. The exhalation should feel the same as a normal exhalation during regular breathing, with no aspirated sound.

BAHYA KUMBHAKA—OUTER RETENTION

Bahya kumbhaka translates as "external breath retention," and it refers to holding the breath after completing an exhalation. Physiologically, it refers to the bottom limit of our expiratory reserve volume. After a complete exhale, we have around 1,200 mL of air left inside our lungs, which means two things:

- There is less oxygen available, so blood oxygen saturation decreases faster.

- The ratio of carbon dioxide to oxygen quickly increases.

Bahya kumbhaka is the most difficult breath retention because it requires holding the breath with only residual reserves for respiratory exchange. But because of the decreased volume in our lungs, our carbon dioxide levels increase much faster, and we experience the effects of hypoxia (low oxygen) and hypercapnia (high carbon dioxide) quicker and more intensely. *Bahya kumbhaka* is generally very difficult for someone who has never practiced it. Holding the breath with empty lungs can give us the feeling of suffocating, evoke panic, and stimulate the fight-or-flight response. But with training and practice, we can use this breath practice to move into deeper states of relaxation and meditation, especially when we are able to incorporate *bahya kumbhaka* with *puraka, rechaka,* and *antara kumbhaka.*

KEVALA KUMBHAKA—SUSPENSION OF BREATHING

Kevala kumbhaka is the suspension of breathing. *Kevala* means "whole," "complete," or "by itself." *Kevala kumbhaka* is said to occur when we are so deep in meditation that the *puraka* and *rechaka* suddenly stop. Then we can maintain the breath-hold indefinitely and obtain the state of *samadhi,* which is the highest level of Patanjali's eightfold path of yoga, the state of bliss and enlightenment. The practice of *kevala kumbhaka* is not the absolute cessation of breathing, but the lengthening of the breath and reduction of how much air we are breathing until it seems as though there is no breath at all. *Kevala kumbhaka* is the highest form of breath retention and breathing less.

There are two primary ways to practice *kevala kumbhaka:*

- **Lengthening the four parts of the breath.** By lengthening the inhalation, holding the in-breath, exhaling, and holding the out-breath, all for as long as we can, we extend one breath cycle to its maximum length. But most people can't do this for more than one cycle, so instead, we find the maximum length of each part of the breath that we can maintain for the longest time.

- **Reducing our tidal volume.** If the normal tidal volume (see page 28) is around 500 mL, then reducing it to 150 to 250 mL while maintaining the same respiratory rate will give us the benefits of *kevala kumbhaka* and breathing less. I find this second way of practicing *kevala kumbhaka* much more challenging and much harder to maintain.

ENERGETIC LOCKS— THE *BANDHAS*

Breath retention is often accompanied by yogic muscular locks called *bandhas*. A *bandha* is a type of energetic gate that regulates the flow of energy. *Bandhas* became very popular with certain yoga practices like ashtanga vinyasa, Baptiste yoga, and power yoga. This gave rise to the invention of many new nontraditional *bandhas*, like *hasta bandha* (hand lock) and *pada bandha* (foot lock). Traditionally, as taught in the ancient yoga literature, there are just four *bandhas*, with the fourth, the *maha* (great) *bandha*, being the combination of the other three *bandhas* practiced together. *Bandha* means "to bind or lock," as in to prevent movement.

I think the majority of yoga practitioners have greatly misunderstood the energetic and physical aspects of the *bandhas*. And it makes sense. Very little is written in the ancient text about how the *bandhas* work. In the *Hatha Yoga Pradipika, bandhas* are meant to "act like safety valves in the human system." Anyone who looks to these ancient texts for explanations of what does what and why is going to find mostly rhetorical claims of the *bandhas* doing magical things, like, "He who constantly practices *uddiyana bandha* as taught by his guru, and as it occurs in a natural way, becomes young though he may be old," as stated in the *Hatha Yoga Pradipika*. And while we see postulations like this relating to what the many practices of yoga can do, we shouldn't discount the value of the practice or the ancient wisdom that has allowed them to endure for so long. I do believe that the *bandhas* have the ability to regulate and control the flow of energy. There are also several physiological benefits to be gained from practicing them together with certain *pranayama* techniques, as you'll see later in this section.

BANDHAS—ENERGETIC LOCKS

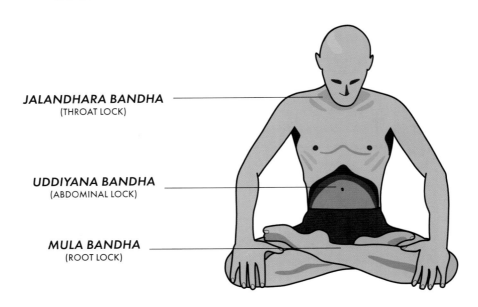

JALANDHARA BANDHA
(THROAT LOCK)

UDDIYANA BANDHA
(ABDOMINAL LOCK)

MULA BANDHA
(ROOT LOCK)

MULA BANDHA—ROOT LOCK

We'll start at the base with the root lock, known as *mula bandha* (*mula* translates as "root"). *Mula bandha* is used to regulate the downward flow of energy called *apana* and is associated with *muladhara,* the root *chakra.* Energetically, *mula bandha* helps us feel grounded and safe. We engage *mula bandha* by lifting the muscles of the pelvic floor, specifically the levator ani, which is located around the perineum, the space between the anus and genitals. This action is similar to a Kegel exercise and is often confused with squeezing the anus.

In the physical *asana* practice, engaging *mula bandha* is sometimes taught as a way to stabilize the pelvis and the core. Personally, I don't find any advantages to lifting my pelvic floor while practicing, although maybe it does help some practitioners. *Mula bandha* is connected to the other two *bandhas* through a continuous line of muscle and fascia known as the deep front line. Many actions and movements create some synergistic engagement of the pelvic floor muscles. For certain types of pelvic floor dysfunctions, as well as for women who recently gave birth or are about to give birth, exercising the *mula bandha* can be beneficial for strengthening the pelvic floor, especially if it is weak. However, continuously engaging *mula bandha* for an hour or more a day for months or years can create lots of problems for most people, especially women. Chronically squeezing the pelvic floor creates overly strong and overly tight muscles. While strength and tightness might not be a problem when it comes to the gluteal muscles, they definitely can be when it comes to the pelvic floor. I had an anatomy teacher who referred to the pelvic floor as the pelvic funnel because it's more like a funnel with things passing through it; therefore, we want these muscles to be supple and elastic. A tight pelvic floor can lead to constipation, hemorrhoids, difficulty or pain while urinating, lower back pain, pain during sex for women, and severe complications during childbirth.

I have a student who was a serious ashtanga vinyasa practitioner for years and would engage *mula bandha* every day during her yoga practice. Because of her overly tight pelvic floor, several muscles in her pelvic floor tore during childbirth, causing debilitating problems and chronic pelvic pain. She is even part of a support group with several other women who had the same complications during labor due to practicing *mula bandha.* The purpose of providing this information is not to say that *mula bandha* is bad or good; I'm saying it's not appropriate or necessary for everyone and should be practiced cautiously with an understanding of why you are practicing it and the effects that your method of practice has on your body.

When approaching any practice, we should be aware of the different ways it is taught and utilized and why, along with all the potential effects. *Mula bandha* is generally taught very differently with *pranayama* than it is with *asana.* In *pranayama, mula bandha* is used as the "seat" of the inhalation to create an energetic anchor as the energy flows upward. During *puraka,* the practitioner gently engages *mula bandha* and releases it during *rechaka* to allow the *apana* energy to release freely. It's important to note that *mula bandha* is not engaged the entire time, as is often taught during an *asana* class.

During the breath sequences covered in Section 5, we will not be practicing *mula bandha.* However, as we engage *uddiyana bandha, mula bandha* might also engage slightly because they are fascially connected.

UDDIYANA BANDHA—ABDOMINAL LOCK

Uddiyana bandha is the abdominal lock. It is sometimes called the upward flying lock because *uddiyana* means "to rise upward" or "to fly up." However, I think it should be called the vacuum lock because of how the *bandha* is engaged. Energetically, *uddiyana bandha* is related to *udana vayu* (see page

80) and helps regulate energy traveling up the center channel of the body. It is also related to the third *chakra, manipura,* which is our center of power, will, vitality, and *agni* (inner fire) and which we can increase by practicing this lock. Physically, *uddiyana bandha* works to strengthen our deep core muscles and diaphragm, helps with gastric motility, stimulates the visceral organs, and moves lymph fluid, which helps remove toxins and strengthen the immune system.

Note: Because of the strong internal pressure *uddiyana bandha* places on the organs, you shouldn't practice *uddiyana bandha* if you are pregnant or have severe gastrointestinal problems.

This *bandha* can be engaged in almost any position. However, it's easiest to learn from a kneeling or standing tripod position, where we place our hands on our knees and lean forward with a neutral spine. This position allows gravity to help fully relax the stomach, making it easier to expand our rib cage to get the maximum lift and engagement from the *bandha.*

To perform *uddiyana bandha,* exhale completely and hold the breath. Lift your belly inward and upward as you pull your navel toward your spine. Trying to inhale with empty lungs without drawing in air creates suction. The diaphragm contracts and the rib cage expands, but because the internal pressure is lower and no air is coming in to equalize the pressure, the stomach is sucked inward. (The result is similar to what it's like when we suck in our cheeks to make a fish face.) *Uddiyana bandha* is almost always practiced with *jalandhara bandha* because *jalandhara bandha* helps reduce the pressure felt in the throat.

During *pranayama, uddiyana bandha* is always practiced during *bahya kumbhaka* (outer retention), which is essential for being able to do the lock. Some yoga teachers teach this *bandha* during *asana* while breathing, but in this case, *uddiyana bandha* really just refers to the way the belly is pulled in and shouldn't be confused with the *pranayama* practices that we will do.

JALANDHARA BANDHA—THROAT LOCK

Jalandhara bandha is the throat lock. *Jal* means "net," and *dhar* is the flow of ambrosia, referring to controlling the flow of energy rising up the *nadis. Jalandhara* is linked with the throat *chakra, vishuddha,* which has to do with expression, purification, and communication. *Jalandhara* works to stimulate the vagus nerve, which controls the parasympathetic nervous system (refer to Section 2). Using *jalandhara bandha* with *uddiyana bandha* increases vagal tone. The synergy between these two locks works with *bahya kumbhaka* to lower blood pressure and heart rate and create a deep calming state.

To engage *jalandhara bandha,* tuck your chin toward your chest, lengthen the back of your neck, and contract your throat as though you are swallowing. This *bandha* can also be used with *antara kumbhaka;* however, I find it most helpful when holding *bahya kumbhaka, uddiyana bandha,* and other practices where we increase internal thoracic pressure without inhaling, like *agnisar pranayama* (see page 150).

PRANAYAMA EXERCISES

Now that you have a solid foundation in the physiology and philosophy of the breath practice, we'll move into some basic *pranayama* exercises. The exercises covered in this section are some of the most common and effective *pranayama* practices. It's good to become familiar with each of these practices. Most *pranayama* exercises have a wide array of effects, both emotional and physiological. As you begin to understand these effects fully, you'll be able to make small changes to direct your practice toward a specific intention. Linking the practices will help even more, as we will explore in Section 4.

CONSIDERATIONS FOR PRACTICING *PRANAYAMA*

Breathing exercises are best done on an empty stomach. Having any food in your belly can make some of these exercises uncomfortable. It's important to feel comfortable and supported when doing these exercises. Consider wearing loose or nonrestrictive clothing so your belly is free to expand with minimal effort. Ideally, you want to practice somewhere quiet and comfortable with minimal distractions. As we move into sequencing breathing exercises in Section 5, the intention of your practice will dictate the best time of day to do the practice. If the intention isn't dependent on the time of day, such as breathing to help with sleep, then practicing in the morning is usually best so you feel the benefits throughout the day.

As already discussed, whenever you are seated, you should have your knees slightly lower than your hips to support your spine so that you can breathe properly. If sitting on the floor is too difficult for you to maintain, then do these practices seated in a chair that supports your spine and proper breathing.

When approaching any *pranayama* practice, especially the more rigorous exercises that involve either rapid breathing or long breath-holds, it's important to take an easy approach. The effects of the breath can be intense and come on rapidly. Breathing too fast can trigger panic attacks and other behavioral changes. Holding the breath can cause our blood pressure to drop rapidly and make us pass out. Although the chances of something bad happening are slim, it's always a good idea to test the waters before jumping in headfirst. Some practices are intense and the effects obvious, while others can be more subtle and take time and repetition before we understand how they truly affect us.

Everyone responds differently to these exercises, so if you don't feel what is described, it doesn't necessarily mean that you are doing it wrong. If a practice doesn't feel good, stop and modify so that it makes sense to you. Having a clear intention of your goals for the practice will help guide you to where you should be. Most important, dedicate the time needed to experience the results of the practice and enjoy the process.

THREE-PART BREATHING—*DIRGHA SVASAM PRANAYAMA*

Dirgha svasam pranayama is the three-part yogic breath also known as the complete yogic breath. *Dirgha* (sometimes spelled *deergha*) means "deep" or "long," and *svasam* refers to breathing. This is usually the first of the *pranayama* practices that I teach to my students because it is the basis for any deep breath. It is called "three-part" breathing because it refers to the order in which the three parts of the torso are expanded: lower, middle, and upper. When we inhale, the air moves down the trachea, bronchi, bronchioles, and alveoli, in that order. The lungs expand in every direction, just like a balloon being inflated. We cannot breathe into the bottom of the lungs before we breathe into the top of the lungs; we also cannot technically breathe into the abdomen. The diaphragm separates the thoracic cavity, which contains the lungs, from the abdominal cavity. The cue "breathe into the belly" isn't literal, but expanding the abdomen expands the lower ribs and in turn expands the chest.

Dirgha svasam is the technique of expanding the container. Thinking back to the example of the balloon in a jar (see page 28), we need to expand the jar to put more air into the balloon. *Dirgha svasam* is the system that allows us to expand the capacity of the container. Although air enters the lungs from the top down and the lungs expand equally, when we work to expand the container, we start from the bottom and move upward because it's the most effective way to increase vital capacity.

The general purpose of this breath is to find our maximum inspiratory capacity by utilizing all our muscles of inhalation. *Dirgha svasam* is an excellent practice for strengthening the diaphragm and intercostal muscles as well as stretching the thoracic cavity to help increase our vital capacity. This practice can also be used to bring more awareness to the breath to focus and calm the mind.

As with all *pranayama* exercises, we must maintain good posture (see pages 41 and 42) so that we can fully utilize our diaphragm and accessory breathing muscles. Fully relax the belly. As you inhale, expand your stomach outward; this action creates more space for the visceral organs and enables the diaphragm to move farther downward as it contracts. Relaxing the core also relieves tension around the lower ribs, which allows the rib cage to expand further. At the same time, as you relax the belly, soften the low back and kidney area to enable the back ribs to expand. The inhalation should expand the lower torso 360 degrees in all directions.

Once you reach the maximum expansion of the lower back and stomach, open up into the middle chest and middle back. Inhaling into the chest pulls the lower ribs upward; however, don't let your shoulders or collarbones lift. The natural tendency is to raise the chest upward rather than expand it outward. Lifting the ribs decreases our vital capacity and the maximum expansion of the chest as well as trains our intercostal muscles to work less efficiently. While focusing on the chest, inhale and allow your collarbones to lift. Then try the same inhalation again, but this time, keep your shoulders relaxed and your collarbones stationary so that all the ribs expand outward and upward toward the collarbones. Hopefully, the second breath felt better and more complete. The collarbones anchor the other intercostal muscles to create the lifting action, which allows for more expansion.

The last component is the upper chest and back. Most people tend to lift their collarbones when breathing into the upper chest. Of these three parts of expanding the container, the upper chest has the least effect, and if you fully inhale into the middle chest, you might not see any more expansion. At this part of the breath, you are looking for full expansion of the lungs and torso. Also think about breathing into your upper back and expanding or widening the shoulder blades; this enables you to expand the back intercostals.

We can also do *dirgha svasam* by taking smaller, less full breaths and focusing on the quality of the breath. Most of the energy and effort should be directed toward the lower torso, then the middle chest, and the least effort into the upper chest. There is a tendency to create unnecessary stress when breathing into the upper chest.

We can think of the three parts of the breath as having different ratios. Instead of breathing equally into the belly, chest, and upper chest, we spend more time expanding the stomach and much less time expanding the upper chest. I use the ratio 3:2:1 as a general guideline. For example, a twelve-second inhalation would involve six seconds of expanding the belly, four seconds of expanding the chest, and two seconds of expanding the upper chest. However, when the inhalations get really long, the ratio becomes closer to 3:3:1. The exhalation should be equal through the chest and belly. You can exhale to the natural pause in the exhalation cycle, where the diaphragm comes to its neutral state, or continue exhaling until the lungs are empty by compressing the chest and belly using the muscles of expiration.

In the beginning, it's good to use a ratio when practicing *dirgha svasam* so that you get comfortable with the fullness of the breath. Once you feel comfortable, you can do three-part breathing more intuitively, which will allow you to focus more on the intention of what you are practicing.

The physiological effects of the breath will change depending on how fast you breathe. Because *dirgha svasam* involves deeper, fuller breaths and moving more air, you will likely be breathing very slowly. When we practice faster breathing, even if the breaths are full and deep, we rarely focus on this level of detail. Without adding *kumbhaka* to this practice, you won't see the advantages that come from increasing our carbon dioxide levels. However, the slower, deeper breathing will increase the amount of nitric oxide you are inhaling.

STEPS TO PRACTICE *DIRGHA SVASAM PRANAYAMA*

1	Sit or stand in a good conventional breathing posture with a tall neutral spine. (Optional: Place one hand on your chest and one hand on your stomach to channel awareness.)
2	Using the breath ratio 3:2:1, inhale into the belly and low back for a count of 6.
3	After the count of 6 and the maximum expansion of the belly, side ribs, and low back, inhale into the mid-chest for a count of 4.
4	After the chest is fully expanded, breathe into the upper chest for a count of 2. Keep your shoulders and collarbones neutral and relaxed.
5	Exhale slowly and equally for a count of 12.
6	Repeat. If needed, change the ratio until you find a count that works for you.

DIRGHA SVASAM PRANAYAMA EFFECTS

Increases nitric oxide
Increases vital capacity and expands total lung capacity
Increases inspiratory reserve
Strengthens the diaphragm and inspiratory muscles
Calms and focuses the mind
Increases *sattva* energy, brings about a state of equanimity
Balances the autonomic nervous system, increases ventral vagal complex tone

VICTORIOUS BREATH—*UJJAYI PRANAYAMA*

Ujjayi pranayama means "the victorious breath." It is also referred to as the ocean breath or occasionally as the Darth Vader breath because of the sound it makes. The *ujjayi* breathing technique is commonly used during physical yoga practices and is probably the most well-known and practiced *pranayama* technique among modern yogis. As mentioned earlier, it is often misused and misunderstood. But before we get all anti-*ujjayi* breath or think that most of us are doing *ujjayi pranayama* wrong, I would like to clarify that there isn't a right or wrong way to do any of these breathing exercises. Breathing is a tool that has many purposes; we can't understand the purpose of the tool unless we know how we want to use it. If we have an intention and our chosen tool doesn't accomplish that intention, either we are using the wrong tool or we are using the right tool in the wrong way.

I use this formula in almost everything that I teach or create:

Intention/purpose + action = intended goal/desired outcome

With the consideration of our intention or purpose, we choose a tool (breathing exercise) with the action that gives us the results we desire.

But for this formula to work, we need to understand why we are practicing with this specific tool. We need to know what the tool does, why it does that, what all of its other uses are, and if we use this particular tool in this specific way, will the results bring us toward our desired goal? I say "all of its other uses" because sometimes a tool does exactly what we want it to do, but it might also do some things we don't want it to do. For example, a strong and loud *ujjayi* breath helps focus the mind, but generating the amount of force needed to create this sound takes a lot of effort, which can result in over-breathing. If we understand the effects, then we can change or modify the practice to do what we intend.

While I have expressed that most of the yogis I have encountered who practice *ujjayi* in their *asana* are over-breathing, they aren't doing it wrong if their intention is to breathe deeper and harder than necessary. In many situations, we might want to breathe like this, but if we are not trying to over-breathe and instead wish to conserve and extend energy, then we probably want to choose another technique or modify the way we are practicing *ujjayi pranayama.* It is ironic that most people practicing *ujjayi* in class are over-breathing because *ujjayi* is one of the most effective methods for slowing and regulating the breath. Still, if we take full, deep breaths without dramatically slowing our rate of breathing, it becomes excessive over time.

Ujjayi pranayama is practiced by mildly tightening the throat as you would if you were whispering softly but with your mouth closed. This action constricts the glottis and narrows the airway. The vocal cords are abducted so that there is no phonation of the voice; instead, the sound is soft and breathy. You can practice by opening your mouth and exhaling as though you were trying to fog up a mirror or make a nonvocalized "ha" sound and then closing your mouth and keeping your throat constricted while exhaling with a silent "ha." Once you feel comfortable and can effortlessly create the *ujjayi* breath on the *rechaka* (exhalation), add it to the *puraka* (inhalation).

This is the basic technique; however, *ujjayi* can be practiced in many ways. I like to compare this breath practice to a garden hose. If I take a hose and place my thumb over the opening, I can regulate the pressure and the amount of water that comes out. This regulation works in conjunction with how much I turn the faucet. If I keep it low, I can water a delicate flower without spraying the dirt everywhere or destroying the flower. If I turn it up high, I can blast dead bugs off my car's windshield. My thumb is basically doing the same thing, but varying the water pressure gives me dramatically different results. With all breathing practices, the depth, rate, and force of the breath will change the effects of the practice.

If a teacher tells you to do it louder when practicing *ujjayi* in class, consider it a red flag. Louder isn't bad, and quieter isn't better, but louder means more force, which means a deeper breath. Unless you are very aware of slowing your breathing, you will over-breathe. As we've discussed in depth, over-breathing can have many negative effects, especially if it is done throughout an entire practice. Understanding the intention of the practice and the effects of the breath will always guide you down the right path and dispel confusion.

Let's move into the uses and benefits of *ujjayi.* The sound it makes is called *ajapa* mantra, which means "the unspoken mantra." In meditation and Eastern philosophy, mantras are powerful tools for training and understanding the mind; in fact, the word *mantra* means "tool for the mind." A mantra is a sound or phrase that is repeated over and over. This repetition acts as a vehicle to guide our thoughts back to the present when the mind begins to wander. Mantras also allow us to focus our thoughts, feelings, and emotions so we can move into deeper states of consciousness that empower us to discover our innate wisdom and reach higher states of spiritual awakening. The *ajapa* mantra sound of *ujjayi* is an effective tool for focusing the mind to be present and keeping it from wandering. If we make it louder and more forceful, then it is easier to focus on and more effective for this purpose—but can we achieve this same focus and presence without being loud?

A well-known and highly respected yoga teacher named Mark Whitwell, who was a student of Krishnamacharya, the father of modern yoga, loves to teach a robust and very loud *ujjayi* breath. In his classes, Whitwell comes around and listens for the intensity of students' breath, often getting very close and repeating "louder" until they reach a volume that he finds sufficient, which usually makes the class sound like a Darth Vader convention. The physical yoga practice that he teaches is also very gentle in comparison to most *asana* practices; in his classes, the focus is clearly on the mind and breath and not the physical movements. His method of practice can be done without over-breathing if emphasis is placed on lengthening the *puraka* and *rechaka*. Extending the breath cycle also helps increase our awareness of the breath. Because Whitwell's *asana* practices are physically less demanding than most classes, keeping a very slow, deep, and loud *ujjayi* is attainable, yet can still be quite challenging. Understanding his intention for the breath gives insight into why he teaches it this way.

I would not teach or practice *ujjayi* this way during a physical practice, even though placing so much emphasis on the quality of the breath is a useful tool to stay present. I teach my yoga students to use *ujjayi* to focus their thoughts and stay present, but my approach is different. I ask my students to create the *ujjayi* to regulate the flow of air and listen for the silence of the breath. When we learn to listen for sounds, we also learn to hear the silence between sounds. Listening for silence is more subtle, takes more control and practice, and is more challenging to maintain. Whitwell's technique is much easier for a beginner to practice and understand the intention of the breath. I rarely teach beginners and mostly educate teachers, which is probably why I lean on the more advanced, softer variation of this breath. However, doing a loud and powerful *ujjayi* breath without over-breathing is a very advanced technique. It can be advantageous to start with an *ujjayi* practice that is louder and a bit more intense to learn the power that it has to guide and train the mind, even though it will most likely result in over-breathing. Sustained over-breathing is never ideal when considering the physiological impact, but sometimes the benefit of learning how to be mindful is more valuable for someone who is lacking in this awareness. As we grow in our practice, we can search for the subtleties that come from the natural evolution until we can experience the same mindful presence through a soft or silent *ujjayi* without the detriment of over-breathing.

A strong, loud *ujjayi* has a few different effects on the body compared to the less forceful, quieter variation. Because constricting the airway makes it more challenging to inhale deeply and exhale fully, this breathing technique works to strengthen the diaphragm and accessory respiratory muscles. The increased power of the breath stimulates the sympathetic nervous system and creates *rajas* energy, which builds internal heat, or *agni.* Constricting the glottis and increasing the pressure in the thoracic cavity and throat causes something interesting to happen. Creating a forced exhalation against the glottis as done in the *ujjayi* breath stimulates the vagus nerve. Increasing vagal tone down-regulates the sympathetic nervous system and has a calming effect; it can also decrease our perception of pain.

A forceful *ujjayi* exhalation is similar to the Valsalva maneuver, which is a technique used to increase vagal tone, slow the heart rate, and decrease blood pressure, among many other things. Medical professionals use the Valsalva maneuver to test cardiac function in relation to the autonomic nervous system. The maneuver is done by forcefully exhaling against a closed airway, like when you hold your breath and bear down or you try to clear your ears by pressurizing the eustachian tubes, the canal that connects the middle ear to the upper throat. While deep over-breathing stimulates sympathetic tone, the increased vagal tone helps inhibit the effects by slowing the heart, decreasing blood pressure, and creating a calm, relaxed feeling. It doesn't mean that these opposing effects completely cancel each other out, however. Over-breathing still decreases carbon dioxide levels, decreases cellular respiration via the Bohr effect (see pages 20 to 23), and increases blood alkalinity. But because of the calming effects and slower heart rate that we see with the increased parasympathetic tone, we don't usually notice that we are over-breathing.

Understanding these varying effects is helpful when it comes to using *ujjayi pranayama.* If I increase my breathing without *ujjayi,* then I get the full impact of increased sympathetic tone versus deep breathing while doing *ujjayi pranayama.* I can now choose which effects I want from over-breathing. Of course, if I really want to hyperventilate to become carbon dioxide deficient, it is extremely difficult to do with *ujjayi* since *ujjayi* restricts airflow.

The sound of *ujjayi* has an interesting physiological effect called autonomous sensory meridian response (ASMR), which causes a pleasurable tingling feeling up the spine, scalp, and back of the neck. ASMR is stimulated by soft whispering, repetitive sounds, and several other triggers. It creates mild euphoria and arousal and has been shown to help people who suffer from depression, anxiety, and panic attacks. On YouTube you'll find millions of ASMR videos of people whispering into microphones to create this body tingle and arousal effect. The soft, repetitive sound of *ujjayi* can also stimulate this physiological response. The effects of ASMR are amplified when we practice *ujjayi* and focus on the sound of the breath with the intention of euphoria and arousal. While ASMR is not usually considered when practicing *ujjayi,* it can aid in other practices that aim to increase libido and sexual arousal. I also find that the ASMR effects are present only when we are static in our *pranayama* practice and not usually noticed during a physical exercise.

Ujjayi is a regulatory tool for lengthening the inhalation and exhalation. It allows us to fine-tune the breath and adds an extra level of control that is difficult to regulate with just the respiratory muscles. I usually use some degree of *ujjayi* when practicing long inhalations and exhalations, but because of the softness and low intensity of the breath, the typical *ujjayi* sound is not heard or is heard only by the practitioner. Unless I am using *ujjayi* to build heat, strengthen my respiratory muscles, or increase energy or virility, I try to use only enough force so that I can hear the breath, but someone sitting next to me can't. *Ujjayi,* when practiced softly and slowly, can move us into deep states of relaxation and concentration. Slower breathing increases parasympathetic tone, and the added vagal tone from the Valsalva maneuver inhibits sympathetic tone. The combination of these two physiological effects makes *ujjayi* a great practice for regulating the autonomic nervous system.

STEPS TO PRACTICE *UJJAYI PRANAYAMA*	
1	Begin in any position.
2	Breathe regularly through the nose.
3	Create a gentle constriction of the throat and exhale as if to fog up a mirror or create a silent "ha" sound.
4	Continue a passive inhalation through the nose with a gently forced exhalation out the nose while maintaining the constriction of the throat and the soft "ha" sound.
5	Add the *ujjayi* breath practice to the inhalation.
6	Practice various degrees of intensity. Try to make it as loud as possible, as soft and quiet as possible, and control the breath so it is audible only to you.

UJJAYI PRANAYAMA EFFECTS (FORCED)	UJJAYI PRANAYAMA EFFECTS (SOFT)
Strengthens respiratory muscles (primarily the diaphragm, internal and external intercostals, and rectus abdominis)	Slows and regulates breathing
Increases vagal tone via the Valsalva maneuver (slows heart rate, lowers blood pressure, decreases pain perception, increases physical strength on exertion)	Increases vagal tone via the Valsalva maneuver (slows heart rate, lowers blood pressure, decreases pain perception, increases physical strength on exertion)
Increases sympathetic tone (focus and energy)	Increases parasympathetic tone (calming, restorative)
Decreases carbon dioxide levels (constricts blood vessels and airways, lowers oxygen exchange)	Increases carbon dioxide levels (opens blood vessels and airways, increases oxygen exchange via the Bohr effect)
Increases blood pH (more alkaline) Increases appetite Increases cravings for acid-forming foods	Decreases blood pH (more acidic) Decreases appetite Increases cravings for alkaline-forming foods
The sound helps focus the mind	Listening for silence creates challenge for the advanced practitioner
Increases *rajas* energy, increases internal heat	Increases *sattva* energy, brings about a state of equanimity
ASMR effects (euphoria, arousal)	

EQUAL RATIO BREATHING—*SAMA VRITTI PRANAYAMA*

Sama vritti is a breathing pattern in which the inhalation and exhalation are equal in duration as well as intensity. Equal ratio breathing can be extended to include the *kumbhakas* (outer and inner retention), which is also called box breathing, square breathing, or four-part breathing. To avoid confusion, I will refer to the equal ratio breathing of the inhalation and exhalation as *sama vritti* and call it box breathing when we add the breath retentions that are equal to the in- and out-breaths.

Sama in Sanskrit means "equal," and *vritti* refers to fluctuations or modifications. Naturally, the exhalation is slightly longer than the inhalation, which gives the breath its natural variations. The mind can be turbulent like an ocean; the ancient yogis believed that if we smoothed the fluctuations of the breath, then the thoughts would follow in equanimity and settle the waves of the mind. Creating equality in the breath is a powerful way to regulate energy, either bringing excessive energy down or raising low energy levels to facilitate a balanced, more *sattvic* state. This balancing of energy works on our emotions to help calm and regulate mood swings or episodes of manic depression. The practice of *sama vritti* balances physical energy to ease agitation and restlessness or lift us out of lethargy, sluggishness, and fatigue.

Sama vritti is a basic breathing exercise in which we use a ratio of 1:1 to match the length of the inhalation and exhalation. For example, if the inhalation is four seconds, the exhalation is also four seconds. We can add *ujjayi pranayama* to help slow and regulate the breath count, which is helpful especially when we lengthen the inhalation and exhalation. When we add the retention for box breathing, the ratio becomes 1:1:1:1.

When we see a two-part breath ratio (e.g., 1:1), as in *sama vritti,* the ratio is always the inhalation and exhalation since these are the minimum components of breathing. In a four-part ratio (e.g., 1:1:1:1), the first number represents the inhalation, the second number is the inward retention, the third number is the exhalation, and the fourth number is the outward retention. For any other ratio, the components will be clarified. For box breathing, if we use four for the ratio, we would inhale for four seconds, hold for four seconds, exhale for four seconds, and hold for four seconds.

To avoid over-breathing in both *sama vritti* and box breathing, we inhale only as much as is necessary. A common mistake is to make every breath a full breath even if the ratio is a low number. For example, if I take a full inhale for four seconds and a full exhale for four seconds, I am breathing 5 liters of air, which equals 37.5 liters of air per minute, when my normal resting rate is 7.5

liters over fifteen breaths per minute. With this example, I am breathing five times as much as usual. Ideally, we want to keep the effort of the inhalation the same as our normal at-rest breath. A four-second inhalation should only partially fill the lungs, and the exhalation shouldn't fully empty the lungs. A longer breath cycle also increases the depth of the inhalation and the force of the exhalation. We do the same thing for box breathing; the only difference is the added retention.

Through my practice, I have noticed that all *pranayama* practices and any type of conscious breathing, even rapid breathing exercises, can settle the mind as long as the intention is clear. What I find interesting with *sama vritti,* which is something I've noticed with many other *pranayama* techniques, is how modern physiology supports the purpose and intention of the claims of the ancient breath practices. Of course, we do see a lot of *pranayama* dogma and unsupported claims of health benefits from various *pranayama* practices. To understand the benefits from the practices we use, we should be able to draw clearly definable lines between Eastern philosophy and Western physiology until both feel like they are saying the same thing but in different languages, and the claims are supported with science.

The purpose of *sama vritti* is to create a sense of equanimity that moves us into a *sattvic* state. *Sattva* is the *guna* that expresses harmony and balance in the body, mind, and spirit. From a Western standpoint, we see *sattva* as the body's condition of homeostasis, where all the systems are in equilibrium. Having high heart rate variability (HRV) shows a healthy and balanced autonomic nervous system, good cardiovascular health, and a high ability to handle stress. High HRV is also an indication of our ability to switch gears quickly, either into more energetic activity or to slow down, rest, and recover. Low HRV is usually associated with chronic stress and poor health. *Sama vritti* has been shown to increase HRV. It's amazing that even a slight variation of our breathing can create noticeable physiological changes. A breath ratio of 5:5 has shown greater improvement in HRV as compared to a ratio of 4:6.[4]

Box breathing acts in the same way to increase HRV. The main physiological benefits from *sama vritti* and box breathing are similar. Changing the length of the retention or the method in which the breathing exercise is practiced alters the physiological and energetic benefits.

Matching the length of the inhalation and exhalation balances the autonomic nervous system, which brings us into a ready state that allows us to quickly up- or down-regulate the nervous system just by changing how we are breathing. We can move into a "go" state and create more sympathetic activation by lengthening the inhalation and shortening the exhalation, or we can move into a "rest" state by extending the exhalation and shortening the inhalation, creating more parasympathetic tone, as discussed earlier. But we can also work to move between the rest, ready, and go states gradually by changing the length of the breath ratio.

Shorter ratios give us more sympathetic activation, and we feel more energized, whereas longer ratios provide us with a more parasympathetic tone, and we feel more relaxed. Overall, *sama vritti* is going to give a balanced autonomic nervous system and a *sattvic* state. Still, we can tip to either side or blend into being balanced and energized or balanced and calm. For example, a ratio of 3:3 is much more energizing than a ratio of 10:10. Also, the longer the ratio, the more *kumbhaka* effects we see, and the benefits that come with breath retention.

My favorite way to use *sama vritti* is to ramp it up or down, although this is not a traditional yogic application of the practice. Ramping up or down the breathing ratios allows us to slowly titrate the effects of the breath practice and use it to gently increase or decrease energy. To ramp up, start with a ratio between 1:1 and 5:5 and increase by one with each breath cycle or every few cycles until you reach your upper limit for the inhalation. Up to 10:10 is entry level, 10:10 to 15:15 is intermediate, and anything over 15:15 is advanced. Let's practice a ramp-up and a ramp-down.

Come into a good posture that supports your breathing and is easy to maintain. Breathe naturally for a few rounds. Start with a breath ratio of 5:5 and increase by 1:1 every round until you reach 10:10, and then go back down by 1:1 and finish where you started. With the same effort of your natural inhalation, inhale for five seconds, and then exhale for five seconds. You can add a soft *ujjayi* breath to help regulate the length of the breath. Inhale for six seconds, exhale for six seconds, inhale for seven seconds, and exhale for seven seconds. As the breath count gets longer, expand the depth and fullness of the breath, increasing the effort. Continue adding by 1:1 until you reach ten seconds, and then work your way back down to a 5:5 ratio. You can ramp up or down box breathing in the same way.

	STEPS TO PRACTICE *SAMA VRITTI PRANAYAMA*
1	Sit or stand in a good conventional breathing posture with a tall neutral spine.
2	Inhale for (4)* seconds and allow a natural pause after the inhalation.
3	Exhale for (4) seconds and allow a natural pause after the exhalation.
4	Repeat (5 to 10 minutes is recommended).

*Numbers in parentheses can change as long as the ratio is 1:1.

	STEPS TO PRACTICE BOX BREATHING
1	Sit or stand in a good conventional breathing posture with a tall neutral spine.
2	Inhale for (4)* seconds.
3	Hold the breath at the top of the inhalation for (4) seconds.
4	Exhale for (4) seconds.
5	Hold the breath after the exhalation for (4) seconds.
6	Repeat (15 minutes is recommended).

*Numbers in parentheses can change as long as the ratio is 1:1.

SAMA VRITTI PRANAYAMA EFFECTS

Balances the autonomic nervous system (regulates blood pressure, heart rate, breathing, and digestion)

Increases HRV (lowers the risk of cardiovascular disease and death, increases cardiovascular fitness, indicates good health)

Decreases chronic stress levels, increases our ability to handle stressful situations

Balances mood and emotions

Supports a *sattvic* state (energetic balance, harmony, spiritual growth)

UNEQUAL RATIO BREATHING—*VISHAMA VRITTI PRANAYAMA*

Vishama vritti pranayama means "unequal breathing," and it refers to any breathing pattern in which there is variation between the lengths of the parts of the breath. The effects generated from *vishama vritti* can vary considerably because changing the ratio of the inhalation to the exhalation or adding a longer or shorter retention alters the physiological effects.

- Generally, the exhalation is twice the inhalation, as seen in the ratio 1:2, meaning that if the inhalation is four seconds, then the exhalation is eight seconds.

- If we add the *antara kumbhaka* (inner retention), the typical retention is four times the inhalation and the exhalation remains double the inhalation, as in the ratio 1:4:2. For example, if the inhalation is four seconds, the inner retention is sixteen seconds and the exhalation is eight seconds.

- The full *vishama vritti* practice also includes the *bahya kumbhaka* (outer retention), which is equal to the length of the inhalation, and we see it as a ratio of 1:4:2:1. So, if the inhalation is four seconds, the inner retention is sixteen seconds, the exhalation is eight seconds, and the outer retention is four seconds.

These are the three breath ratios that are most common in traditional *pranayama* for *vishama vritti,* with 1:2 being the easiest and 1:4:2:1 being the most difficult.

I left out one variation; this is where we skip the *antara kumbhaka* and focus on the *bahya kumbhaka.* This ratio is expressed as 1:2:1, where the inhalation is one, the exhalation is two, and the outer retention is one. This variation is rarely practiced, but working with breathing patterns that focus on lengthening the exhalation has a lot of value, as we'll explore later.

When we practice using these ratios, adding even one second to the inhalation can increase the level of difficulty exponentially. For example, if the inhalation is six seconds, or 6:24:12:6, then the breath cycle is forty-eight seconds long. If we increase the inhalation to seven seconds (7:28:14:7), the breath cycle is fifty-six seconds long. Adding only four seconds to the inhalation and increasing it to ten seconds (10:40:20:10) makes the breath cycle one minute twenty seconds long, almost double the ratio based on six seconds. As with all *pranayama* practices, the longer we maintain the practice, the greater the effects. This is especially true with *vishama vritti* because ultimately it is a *kumbhaka* (breath retention) practice. When practicing *vishama vritti* and trying to find the ratio that works for you, aim to be able to maintain the breath for at least ten minutes before adding another second to the ratio.

Different approaches to *vishama vritti* give us different physiological and emotional effects based on our intention. If we adhere to the 1:4:2:1 ratio and practice it in a way that is easy to maintain, we will feel calm, relaxed, and meditative. If we increase the length of each breath cycle to the point that it is extremely challenging but still maintainable, the feeling of breath hunger will increase quickly and require us to control the response from the sympathetic nervous system mentally. This kind of training has great value in managing anxiety and panic but can also put us into a state of anxiety and panic. Based on our ability to handle the breath practice, we can see a sympathetic response that would come from panicking, or we might have the opposite response with an increase in parasympathetic tone that comes from the increased carbon dioxide levels and our ability to remain calm even when resisting the strong urge to breathe.

The ratio of 1:4:2:1 is great for practicing sustained *kumbhaka*. As I have said, being able to hold a single breath for a long time is great, but we see the most benefits from practicing breath retention over a long period. This specific ratio allows us to prolong the parts of the breath that are easiest to lengthen and shorten the parts that are more difficult to extend. The relationship of respiration to retention is only 3:5, one for inhalation plus two for exhalation, and four for inner retention plus one for outer retention. Because the time we spend inhaling and exhaling is more than half the time we are holding the breath, we can maintain the practice longer, giving us time to recover quickly from the breath-holds while still enabling us to breathe less.

Sustaining this extended breath cycle over a longer period builds up carbon dioxide, increasing cellular respiration and oxygenation of the cells, lowering blood pressure, and slowing the heart. After several rounds of continuous *vishama vritti,* the spleen contracts and releases more red blood cells into the bloodstream, boosting the amount of oxygen-carrying hemoglobin. Prolonged unequal ratio breathing practices also result in the body producing more red blood cells, which improves VO_2 max and athletic performance. The effects of the practice increase when the breath values are higher. A ratio of 3:12:6:3 might not create enough of a demand for the spleen to release more red blood cells, especially if the breath practice feels easy. But if we increase those values to something more challenging, like 7:28:14:7, and start to experience a little breath hunger, then the physiological effects from the practice are much more noticeable.

Of course, building up to this point takes time, and the ratio we choose shouldn't be based on achieving the highest possible numbers, although higher ratios and longer holds come with added health and athletic benefits. Instead, we should aim to find a ratio that is challenging yet sustainable. Practicing longer breath cycles for longer durations builds our tolerance to carbon dioxide, allowing us to retain the breath for much longer before feeling breath hunger. *Vishama vritti,* when practiced within our capabilities, stimulates more parasympathetic tone and *tamasic* energy, bringing us into a relaxed, more meditative state. This *pranayama* practice is great for recovering from exercise and exertion, boosting the immune system, or recovering from illness (although, if it is a respiratory infection, doing the long holds can be challenging).

However, adhering only to this standard ratio dramatically limits our use of the breath. With *vishama vritti,* we can change the length values to whatever serves our purpose. Much of what I have talked about already has to do with how the inhalation and exhalation relate to the effect on our autonomic nervous system and energetic body and how breath retention has a physiological influence on our bodies. If we apply our knowledge of how the different components of the breath affect us, then we can adjust the ratio to guide our intention of whatever practice we are doing.

We see this in techniques like 4-7-8 breathing, which doctors and therapists use to help calm and relax patients experiencing high levels of stress and anxiety. The inhalation is four seconds, the inner retention is seven seconds, and the exhalation is eight seconds. Whenever the exhalation is double the inhalation, the technique is going to stimulate the sympathetic nervous system and create more *tamasic* energy. Adding a short retention slows the breathing even more and allows for a slight increase of carbon dioxide without the practitioner feeling any added stress or breath hunger from the hold that they might experience with a longer retention. The shorter retention is especially helpful if the person is not used to holding their breath and already suffering from anxiety.

If we wanted to focus on working on our *bahya kumbhaka,* we could use a ratio of 1:2:2:4. To increase *rajas* and sympathetic tone to have more energy, we could practice a breath ratio of 4:1, where the inhalation is four times as long as the exhalation. There are so many ways to use the breath just by changing the ratio of these four components. I will give many more examples as we move into the breath sequences in Section 5. However, just using your knowledge of how the breath affects the various systems of the body will give you the tools to modify *vishama vritti* to fit your purpose.

STEPS TO PRACTICE *VISHAMA VRITTI PRANAYAMA*

1   Sit or stand in a good conventional breathing posture with a tall neutral spine.

2   Use the ratio (1:4:2:1)*.

3   Inhale for (4) seconds.

4   Hold the inner retention for (16) seconds.

5   Exhale for (8) seconds.

6   Hold the outer retention for (4) seconds.

7   Repeat as needed (15 minutes is recommended).

*Ratios and numbers in parentheses can be changed to meet the desired intention.

VISHAMA VRITTI PRANAYAMA EFFECTS*

Increases carbon dioxide levels (increases cellular oxygenation, lowers blood pressure, lowers heart rate, opens airways, lowers blood pH)

Increases VO_2 max, increases the amount of circulating red blood cells via splenic contraction and red blood cell production on demand

Increases carbon dioxide tolerance (increasing our ability to hold the breath longer)

Stimulates the parasympathetic nervous system (rest and digest, decreases pain perception)

Supports a *tamasic* state (grounding, deep relaxation, promotes sleep)

*Effects will change based on the breath ratio and breath rate.

SKULL SHINING BREATH—*KAPALABHATI PRANAYAMA*

The *pranayama* practices discussed up to this point focus mainly on slowing the breath and working on breath retention. These next few practices are very similar to each other, only with some minor differences, so they are often confused or mislabeled as different practices. But all three of these *pranayama* practices increase the respiration rate, so they have similar physiological effects. We'll dive deep into this first practice and then cover the differences with the other two, bellows breath and breath of fire.

Kapalabhati means "skull shining breath" or "skull illuminating breath." It is traditionally used in yoga for cleansing the mind and body and increasing energy levels. The rapid physical activation of the core and compression of the visceral organs might have a positive effect on moving lymph fluid and increasing circulation in the abdominal cavity to help cleanse the abdominal organs, which can help strengthen the immune system and detoxify the body.

Kapalabhati pranayama is characterized by a forced exhalation with a passive inhalation through the nose. It is easiest to practice this breath in a cross-legged sitting position with the hips situated higher than the knees, or in a kneeling position. The action of the exhalation is very similar to the inward and upward movement of the belly in *uddiyana bandha* (see page 101), so finding a position that enables this movement with control of the belly is vital to sustaining this breathing exercise.

Our normal resting breath pattern happens in our tidal volume range, with an active inhalation and a passive exhalation. When we inhale, the diaphragm contracts and pulls down to expand the thoracic space and lowers the atmospheric pressure inside the chest, and outside air rushes into the lungs and neutralizes the pressures. When we exhale normally, the diaphragm relaxes and draws up, raising inner thoracic pressure and creating a passive exhalation as we expel the air out of our lungs. *Kapalabhati* works in the opposite way. We move past the limit of our passive exhalation as we exhale into the area of our expiratory reserve volume, or the part of our lungs that we can access only through a forced exhalation. Forcing exhalation engages the core and intercostal muscles that contract the torso to lower the atmospheric pressure inside the chest so that when we relax, the torso naturally expands and the inhalation is passive. As we exhale with this technique, we pull the belly in with a fast, forceful contraction that rapidly forces the air out of the lungs. A common mistake is actively inhaling after the forced exhalation and filling the lungs more than intended.

A forced exhalation with a passive inhalation moves about 500 to 750 mL of air per respiration, or roughly half of our expiratory reserve volume plus a portion of our tidal volume. If we add an active inhalation, we can easily double the amount of air and breathe more than we intend to. Passive inhalation takes practice because it's not a breathing pattern that we are used to. *Bhastrika* and breath of fire have active inhalations, and I'll discuss why we might choose to do those practices over *kapalabhati* next.

Kapalabhati is a rapid breathing exercise, with each breath being around a second or less. We are restricted in how fast we can do this practice because we have to wait for the passive inhalation, which acts as a nice regulator to the speed at which we practice. When you first start to practice this technique, it's good to go slower, with each breath cycle being one to two seconds long, so that you can feel the active exhalation and passive inhalation. You should hear the sound of the exhalation but not the inhalation. Once you feel comfortable, speed up the breath to a point where you can maintain proper technique and sustain the practice for at least a minute. It's easy to lose the breath and the rhythm if you go too fast. You want to make each breath smooth and even with a strong contraction of the core with each exhalation.

Kapalabhati pranayama practice is a mild controlled hyperventilation. We see very different physiological effects than we experience with breath retention and hypoventilation. For example, breathing less increases the carbon dioxide in our bloodstream, which raises our blood acidity, enabling better oxygen delivery to the cells via the Bohr effect. As discussed earlier, hemoglobin (the part of the red blood cells that carries oxygen) needs a slightly more acidic environment to release oxygen to the cells. I reiterate this now because most literature about *kapalabhati* says that the practice increases oxygen to the brain and body, which goes along with the common myth that breathing more means more oxygen. As you've learned, the science says the opposite; breathing less brings more oxygen to the brain and body.

Kapalabhati is a very mild form of hyperventilation that is easy to sustain without feeling light-headed and dizzy like we usually would from breathing too fast. Because we are moving much less air per respiration, we don't breathe off as much carbon dioxide as we would if we were taking large breaths but keeping the same breathing rate. The faster breathing still expels carbon dioxide and hydrogen atoms, which makes our blood more alkaline, constricts our blood vessels, narrows our airways, and stimulates the sympathetic nervous system. The sympathetic nervous system is our fight-or-flight response or mobilization response. Our blood vessels constrict and our heart rate and blood pressure rise so that more blood can be sent to the extremities to help mobilize us. The upper airways constrict to retain some of the carbon dioxide as we breathe faster as well as increase the pressure in the lungs to force more air into the alveolar sacs.

As I have said, the autonomic nervous system is not an all-or-nothing system; instead, the sympathetic or parasympathetic tone is titrated as needed through the release of epinephrine and norepinephrine and can be controlled by the way we breathe. *Kapalabhati* is a fantastic practice for stimulating the sympathetic nervous system and creating more *rajas* energy to motivate us toward achieving our goals and create focus and purpose. Faster breathing increases our metabolism and burns calories. The forced exhalation is also a really good action for toning the core and developing neuromuscular response from the abdominal muscles to rapidly stabilize the core, which can benefit us in sports and dynamic exercises.

The rapid breathing from *kapalabhati* creates a mild deficiency of carbon dioxide. Our drive to breathe comes from two factors: lack of oxygen, which we rarely experience because it is difficult to lower SpO_2 unless we hold our breath for a long time, and the buildup of carbon dioxide in our blood. Primarily, it is the increased carbon dioxide levels that urge us to take our next breath. By breathing rapidly, we expel more carbon dioxide than normal and become hypocapnic, which means having low carbon dioxide. The deficiency of carbon dioxide enables us to hold our breath for much longer while carbon dioxide slowly builds back up and urges us to breathe again. *Kapalabhati* does create hypocapnia, but because the breathing is more regulated, it is not as effective as *bhastrika pranayama.* However, this is still something we should be aware of as we practice this technique.

Note: Because of the forceful abdominal contractions, you should not do this breath practice if you are pregnant or you have gastrointestinal problems.

STEPS TO PRACTICE *KAPALABHATI PRANAYAMA*

1	Sit in a kneeling or cross-legged position, with the hips higher than the knees and a tall neutral spine.
2	Allow the diaphragm to relax after a passive exhalation and before a normal inhalation.
3	Forcefully exhale out the nose by contracting the core and pulling the belly in toward the spine. You should hear an audible "puff" sound through the nose as you exhale.
4	Relax the abdominal muscles for a passive, noncontrolled inhalation through the nose. The inhalation should be silent.
5	Start at a rate you can sustain for at least 1 minute, aiming for an exhalation every 1 to 2 seconds.
6	Speed up to a rate you can sustain for at least 1 minute while keeping a strong, forceful exhalation and a smooth, passive inhalation. Aim for an exhalation every 0.5 to 1 second.
7	Repeat 1- to 2-minute cycles for a minimum of 3 to 5 rounds. Depending on the intention of the practice, it's good to follow up with a type of *kumbhaka* practice.

KAPALABHATI PRANAYAMA EFFECTS

Decreases carbon dioxide levels (constricts blood vessels, increases blood pressure, increases peripheral perfusion, constricts upper airways)

Activates the sympathetic nervous system (mobilization response, increases energy, increases metabolism, decreases digestive functions, increases pain perception)

Strengthens and tones abdominal muscles and intercostal muscles, increases abdominal activation and core response time

Increases blood alkalinity (temporarily increases joint mobility)

Carbon dioxide deficiency enables longer breath retention

Increases *rajas guna* (more energy, focus, drive to achieve goals)

Stimulates visceral organs (increases lymph circulation and detoxification)

BELLOWS BREATH—*BHASTRIKA PRANAYAMA*

Bhastrika means "bellows" in Sanskrit, and it describes the dynamic filling and emptying of the lungs, like a blacksmith using a bellows to stoke a fire. *Bhastrika* is similar to *kapalabhati,* except there is a forced inhalation as well as a forced exhalation. Imagine how pumping a bellows forces air in and out. This breath practice is traditionally used to ignite our inner *agni* (digestive fire) and boost energy levels. Raising our blood pH levels increases appetite and, when followed by breath retention, aids in detoxification and elimination. *Bhastrika* creates a lot of *rajas* energy, and similar to *rajas,* this powerful practice can quickly exhaust itself, so we must be aware of how we use and manage the practice.

Energetically, *bhastrika* is focused around the third *chakra* at the navel, which represents self-esteem, willpower, and sense of purpose. Most of these qualities center on having a positive view of ourselves, which fosters healthy social engagement with others. When we have an imbalance or dysfunction in this area, we become introverted, insecure, and anti-social. Usually, these feelings of repression are a sign of a chronically overstimulated dorsal vagal complex, which is responsible for the freeze response. *Bhastrika* is a powerful tool to suppress the dorsal vagal tone and help mobilize us by balancing the nervous system or to increase our energy when we are in a low or balanced state.

To practice *bhastrika,* we start in the same sitting posture as we would with *kapalabhati* so that we can easily expand and contract the belly. With *bhastrika,* we move approximately 1,000 to 1,500 mL of air per breath depending on the force of our respirations, or two to three times as much as we would in normal breathing. Each breath is exaggerated and is well controlled by the abdominal muscles and diaphragm. On the inhalation, forcefully push your belly outward as you partially fill the lungs. The breath is deeper than a normal breath but not as deep as a full inhalation. On the exhalation, pull your belly in toward the spine and hollow out your stomach, similar to the forced exhalation in the *kapalabhati* technique. The inhalation and exhalation should be audible as the air rushes in and out of your nostrils. The inhalation and exhalation should match in length and intensity and should be as smooth as possible while keeping the pumping action of the stomach. The speed of this breath will vary depending on our focus or intention. Breathing slower usually results in a deeper breath and more attention around the contractions of the core. Faster breathing expels more carbon dioxide but also takes more practice and coordination to keep the breath smooth and consistent. The typical range for *bhastrika* is one to two breaths per second.

Bhastrika pranayama requires the most effort of these three rapid breathing exercises and is the hardest to maintain. With this breath, we can quickly stimulate the sympathetic nervous system to increase our energy levels, boost our metabolism, increase our appetite, and get ourselves moving.

The contractions of the core strengthen and tone the belly, and the rapid, forced inhalations strengthen the diaphragm. The movement of the stomach stimulates the abdominal organs. However, the activation of the sympathetic nervous system suppresses gastric mobility and increases colonic tone. Traditionally, this practice is followed by breath retention. When we hold the breath after stimulating the abdominal organs with *bhastrika,* the breath retention allows carbon dioxide to build back up to suppress the sympathetic nervous system and activate the parasympathetic nervous system, which boosts digestion and lowers colonic tone for elimination. One of the advantages of *bhastrika,* and one of the main reasons I employ this rapid breathing practice, is to quickly expel a large amount of carbon dioxide and create a carbon dioxide–deficient environment.

As discussed with *kapalabhati,* the more hypocapnic we are, the longer we can hold our breath before having the urge to breathe. Because carbon dioxide levels take a while to build back up when we are holding our breath, we utilize more of the oxygen in our blood, and this lowers our SpO_2 levels. Less oxygen in the blood creates more of a demand for red blood cells and stimulates their production, similar to the effects of high-altitude training (see pages 36 and 37).

Note: Because of the forceful abdominal contractions, you should not do this breath practice if you are pregnant or you have gastrointestinal problems.

STEPS TO PRACTICE *BHASTRIKA PRANAYAMA*

1	Sit in a kneeling or cross-legged position, with the hips higher than the knees and a tall neutral spine.
2	Inhale forcefully through the nose as you expand the belly outward.
3	Exhale forcefully through the nose by contracting the core and pulling the belly in toward the spine.
4	Respirations should be smooth and even, and you should hear the in and out breath.
5	Repeat 1- to 2-minute cycles for a minimum of 3 to 5 rounds. Depending on the intention of the practice, it's good to follow up with a *kumbhaka* practice.

BHASTRIKA PRANAYAMA EFFECTS

Decreases carbon dioxide levels (constricts blood vessels, increases blood pressure, increases peripheral perfusion, constricts upper airways)

Activates the sympathetic nervous system (mobilization response, increases energy, increases metabolism, decreases digestive functions, increases pain perception)

Strengthens and tones abdominal muscles, intercostal muscles, and diaphragm

Increases blood alkalinity (increases appetite)

Carbon dioxide deficiency enables longer breath retention

Increases *rajas guna* (more energy, focus, drive to achieve goals)

Stimulates visceral organs (increases lymph circulation and detoxification)

Helps with digestion and elimination when followed by breath retention

BREATH OF FIRE—*AGNI PRAN PRANAYAMA*

Breath of fire is a fundamental *pranayama* technique used in kundalini yoga and is a foundational part of many different kundalini *kriyas* (exercises). Yogi Bhajan, who brought kundalini yoga to the West, suggested that people should practice breath of fire until they build up to a continuous thirty-one minutes to burn away karma and disease, as well as to receive many other health benefits. In general, most people practice breath of fire for rounds of only one to three minutes.

Bhastrika and *kapalabhati* are both often incorrectly referred to as "breath of fire" even though they use different techniques. The main differences with the breath of fire are the way we breathe, the speed of the respirations, and the amount of air moved per respiration. The inhalation and exhalation are active but gentler and less forced. There is no intense contraction of the core like we see in *bhastrika* and *kapalabhati;* instead, the effort of breathing is more balanced between the belly and solar plexus area. The breath is smooth and shallow, approximately two to three breaths per second. It should feel like you are moving the air from the upper respiratory system rather than deep in the lungs. The power of the breath comes more from the movement of the diaphragm and intercostal muscles and less from the stomach muscles. The belly should remain soft and relaxed during the practice. Each breath should move about the same amount of air or even a little less than normal breathing, roughly 500 mL. There is an audible breath through the nose during the respirations, which should sound smooth and even on the inhalation and exhalation. Because there is not a focus on the forceful contraction of the core, many people starting this practice do paradoxical breathing, where the belly draws in on the inhalation and out on the exhalation. With breath of fire, we want to maintain healthy breathing habits, allowing the ribs to rise on the inhalation without lifting the shoulders or collarbones and the belly to expand like we would if breathing normally. The stomach should pull in slightly as it follows the movement of the chest.

Breath of fire, like the other faster breathing exercises, stimulates the sympathetic nervous system, increases *rajas* energy, and decreases carbon dioxide levels in the blood. So, with this breath, we experience most of the energetic and physiological effects that we do with *kapalabhati* and *bhastrika*. Breath of fire is generally faster than *bhastrika* and *kapalabhati*, and because it takes less effort, it is easier to sustain. With breath of fire, we can generally continue the practice longer to create more sympathetic tone, increase stamina, and strengthen our upper respiratory muscles. This breath also moves a lot of physical and emotional energy through the body, which can result in significant emotional release. Some therapists use breathing exercises like this with their patients to stimulate emotional breakthroughs.

With any breath practice that focuses on rapid breathing, if we do it long enough, we will eventually breathe off a significant amount of carbon dioxide and begin to feel the hypocapnic effects, like increased heart rate, light-headedness, and dizziness. Over-breathing can cause calcium levels in the blood to drop, which can result in tingling or numbness in the hands, feet, face, and belly. It can also cause carpopedal spasms, where the hands and feet cramp. These sensations are harmless and will resolve themselves after we return to regular breathing or after a few breath-holds where we increase the carbon dioxide levels.

In people who have a history of anxiety and panic disorders, doing any type of rapid breathing can trigger a panic attack. Panic attacks often lead to rapid breathing as a coping mechanism to deal with fear and anxiety. Increasing our respirations is a natural response to the sympathetic nervous system's fight-or-flight response. However, when someone starts to hyperventilate from a panic attack, the effects of over-breathing can make the situation much worse. During the attack, it can feel like we aren't getting enough air, so we breathe faster, which makes us feel dizzy, light-headed, confused, and even more scared. Someone who has experienced this a few times will start to feel the sensations of a panic attack coming on from doing rapid breathing exercises.

Breath of fire, *bhastrika,* and *kapalabhati* are mild enough practices that they don't often trigger panic attacks. The fact that these exercises are gentle and controlled enables people with anxiety and panic disorders to learn how to control their anxiety. Since they can initiate the breathing exercise from a calm and relaxed state, control its intensity, and stop the breath, it helps them learn how to manage the breath when a real panic attack comes on and, in some cases, prevent the episode from happening altogether.

The faster and deeper the breath is, the more likely it is to trigger a panic attack. Later, I will discuss some open-mouth hyperventilation techniques that have a high probability of triggering panic attacks in people who are prone to them. A lot of research has been done on the breathing technique taught by Wim Hof, and this rapid breathing followed by long *kumbhaka* holds has been shown to significantly help people who have panic disorders, depression, and other behavioral maladies.

STEPS TO PRACTICE BREATH OF FIRE

1	Start in a comfortable seated or kneeling position.
2	Rapidly breathe in and out of the nose, 2 to 3 breaths per second.
3	The power of the breath should come from the solar plexus and upper belly area.
4	Keep the stomach soft and relaxed.
5	The breath should be rhythmic and continuous with an equal inhalation and exhalation.
6	Continue for 1 to 3 minutes, repeating for 3 to 5 rounds.

Depending on the intention of the practice, it's good to follow up with a *kumbhaka* practice (see pages 96 to 98).

BREATH OF FIRE EFFECTS

Decreases carbon dioxide levels (constricts blood vessels, increases blood pressure, increases peripheral perfusion, constricts upper airways)

Activates the sympathetic nervous system (mobilization response, increases energy, increases metabolism, decreases digestive functions, increases pain perception)

Increases blood alkalinity (increases appetite)

Carbon dioxide deficiency enables longer breath retention

Increases *rajas guna* (more energy, focus, drive to achieve goals)

Improves mood and affect

ALTERNATE NOSTRIL BREATHING—
NADI SHODHANA PRANAYAMA

Nadi shodhana is a cleansing breath practice used to balance the *ida* and *pingala nadis,* or the subtle energetic currents of the mind and body. In Sanskrit, *shodhana* means "purification," and *nadi,* as previously discussed, refers to the *prana* channels that flow throughout the body.

This practice uses alternate nostril breathing and *mudras* to circulate *prana,* release energetic stagnation, and restore harmony to any subtle body imbalances. The imbalances being regulated can be emotional, physical, or spiritual. The main focus of this practice is to bring us back into a *sattvic* state. Physically, alternating the intention through the breath and touch can help bring balance to the left and right hemispheres of the brain. When the hemispheres are balanced, aspects of the mind, like intuition and intelligence, come together so that we can see things less subjectively and experience a more accurate perception of reality.

Spiritually, the practice both grounds and elevates our state of consciousness, allowing us to feel rooted so that we can expand our awareness without losing reality and yet still grow beyond the limits of perception. Think of this as the balancing aspects represented by the qualities of *udana vayu* and *apana vayu,* where we are grounded in our sense of self without being attached to identity and conscious of our interconnected nature without discarding ourselves in the process. Emotionally, this breathing exercise can calm feelings of anxiety, fear, agitation, and restlessness or help pull us out from feeling down, lethargic, or unhappy. Whatever tools we use to control our emotions, they are still tools—meaning, for the tool to be useful, we need to have a purpose for using that tool and use it in a way that is guided by our intention.

Emotions come from our perception of the world, how we fit into this world, how we think other people are treating us, how we feel about ourselves, and how we compare ourselves to other people. Essentially, we experience everything that we know or encounter as an emotion. All of our memories are emotional; even if we were indifferent to an experience, we remember that event apathetically, and apathy is an emotion. Therefore, to change how we feel, whether that's nervous, overly excited, depressed, lonely, or whatever, we have to change how we perceive the situation and how we see ourselves as part of that situation.

But if being happy was as simple as choosing to be happy, then one in six people wouldn't be on antidepressant medications, and nobody would suffer from depression. We can't just change our minds and decide not to be afraid or sad (at least most people can't), because we are not directly in control of our minds. The best we can be is indirectly in control. We can train the mind to respond and react to a new situation. We can practice removing preferences and conditions that we think we need to be happy. We can repair unhealthy relationships with ourselves and with others. We can do meditation practices like *vipassana* that help us understand the ultimate truth and reality of existence. And we can use the breath and our intention to guide our emotions, regulate our nervous system, and change our physiological chemistry. Because our emotions are chemicals experienced as feelings and our breath can alter these chemicals, the breath is one of the most effective tools for managing our emotional well-being.

Nadi shodhana has four powerful components that make it an extremely useful tool for creating balance in the mind and body and guiding the mind back to a pure, harmonious state. These components are

- The breath
- Our intention
- *Mudras*
- Visualization

The *mudras* and visualization are really just vehicles to guide the intention. The intention for the practice should be more personal than a general intention to purify or balance the mind and body, although there is nothing wrong with that intention. When setting our intention, we should take a few moments to look inward, feel the natural breath, and observe our emotions and any imbalances we might notice. Once we understand our current state, we set the intention to move toward the feeling of the emotion that will create a sense of balance and harmony. We want to focus on the energetic feeling or emotion rather than on words or something intellectual because emotions are not always rational, and intellectual thoughts will not help us very much.

Once we have our intention, we select *mudras* as a representation of our intention and as a tool to focus and manifest our intention through the practice. Traditionally, two specific *mudras* are used for this practice, but if you have another *mudra* that guides your intention, then it's okay to use that *mudra* instead.

- The left hand is used for *jnana mudra,* the *mudra* of knowledge and wisdom. *Jnana mudra* is also commonly used with meditation. To hold this *mudra,* you place the index finger at the base of the thumb to create a small circle and extend the other three fingers. Alternatively, you can touch the tip of the thumb and index finger together, like making the OK sign. The thumb represents the universal consciousness, and the index finger represents the individual self, soul, or ego. Linking the two represents connection or oneness with the supreme reality. The other three fingers portray the nature of the *sattva, rajas,* and *tamas gunas.* The philosophy is that by transcending the physical energies of nature, we can reach the ultimate reality.

- The right hand creates *Vishnu mudra,* or the *mudra* of universal balance. Vishnu is the Hindu deity responsible for protecting and preserving humanity and keeping the universe in balance. To make this *mudra,* you fold the index and middle fingers against the palm and extend the other three fingers.

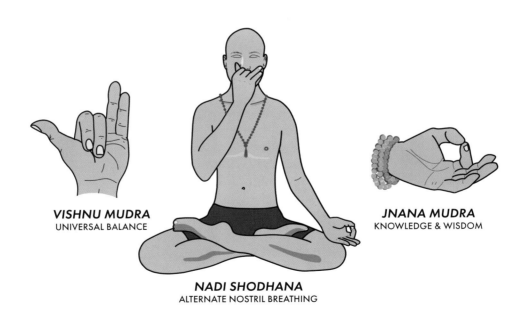

VISHNU MUDRA
UNIVERSAL BALANCE

JNANA MUDRA
KNOWLEDGE & WISDOM

NADI SHODHANA
ALTERNATE NOSTRIL BREATHING

To put *nadi shodhana* into practice, start in a seated position and rest your left hand on your left knee in *jnana mudra.* Place your right hand in *Vishnu mudra* and lightly close off your right nostril with your right thumb.

Alternatively, you can place your index and middle fingers on your forehead while using your thumb and index finger to alternate blocking the nares. Traditionally, *nadi shodhana* was always done with the right hand because this was the hand that touched the face. In India, the left hand was used for cleaning oneself after using the toilet, and touching one's face with one's left hand was considered unclean. However, I don't think it matters which hand we use for the practice nowadays. Most people wipe with their dominant hand, and most are right-handed. Hopefully, everyone washes their hands after doing their business.

Nadi shodhana alternates the flow of the breath between the right and left nostrils. Start by inhaling through your left nostril because the left side is the *ida* side, which represents receptivity. At the top of the breath, close off the left nostril with your ring finger, release the right nostril, and exhale out the right side. Begin the next round by inhaling through the right side and exhaling out the left. With each respiration, alternate between the two nostrils: inhale through the right side, exhale out the left side, inhale through the left side, exhale out the right side, and so on. The nasal cycle (see page 23) and excess mucus can make it difficult to alternate. It's important not to push too hard when closing off the nares.

It's not just the breath that you are moving, but energy, guided by your intention with the breath. While most people don't teach visualization with *nadi shodhana,* I find visualizing the *prana* flowing up and down the *ida* and *pingala nadis* with each breath very helpful in using the intention to create balance. Touching the right and left nostrils also helps bring sensation and awareness to the two hemispheres of the mind.

The force, depth, and rate of our breathing in *nadi shodhana* can change based on our intention. The breath can be natural and follow our resting tidal volume breath, or we can add *ujjayi* (see pages 108 to 113) and *kumbhaka* (see pages 96 to 98) to the practice. Changing the qualities of the breath can significantly affect the energetic and physiological benefits that we experience from the practice. When we practice *nadi shodhana,* we need to choose the quality of breath that complements our intention. Naturally, *nadi shodhana* helps regulate how much air we can move because we are breathing through only one nostril at a time, essentially cutting in half the amount of air we take in. So, combining breath of fire with *nadi shodhana* can increase our *rajas* energy and stimulate the sympathetic nervous system while limiting how much carbon dioxide we expel. This breath practice is a powerful tool for hitting the reset button and restoring balance to the mind and body. But its ability to be combined with almost any other *pranayama* exercise gives it unlimited possibilities to bring about a better state of well-being.

STEPS TO PRACTICE NADI SHODHANA PRANAYAMA

1	Sit in a chair, in a kneeling position, or cross-legged, with your hips higher than your knees and a tall neutral spine.
2	Place the back of your left hand on your left leg or in your lap in *jnana mudra*.
3	With the right hand in *Vishnu mudra*, or two fingers on your forehead, gently close off your right nostril with your thumb.
4	Inhale through the left nostril.
5	Release the right nostril and close the left nostril.
6	Exhale out the right nostril.
7	Repeat the cycle, inhaling through the right side and exhaling through the left side, while alternating closing off each nostril.
8	As you inhale through the left nostril, visualize the energy moving up the left side of your spine or the *ida nadi*. As you exhale, visualize the energy moving down the right side of your spine or the *pingala nadi*.
9	Throughout the practice, you can visualize the center, *sushumna* channel, slowly filling as you create balance between the *ida* and *pingala nadis*.
10	Repeat the cycle—in left, out right, in right, out left—for 5 to 10 minutes or longer if desired.

NADI SHODHANA PRANAYAMA EFFECTS

Balances our emotional well-being
Cleanses the *ida* and *pingala nadis*
Balances the left and right hemispheres of the brain
Regulates and balances the autonomic nervous system
Supports a *sattvic* state (energetic balance, harmony, spiritual growth)
Regulates the amount of air we can move per breath

INTERRUPTED BREATHING—
VILOMA PRANAYAMA

Viloma pranayama is a type of breath practice where the respirations are interrupted by periods of *kumbhaka. Viloma* is Sanskrit for "against the fur," like petting a dog or cat in the wrong direction. The name suggests that breath is moving against the natural current by breaking the flow of air. There are three variations of *viloma pranayama:*

- *Viloma* 1: interruption of the inhalation
- *Viloma* 2: interruption of the exhalation
- *Viloma* 3: interruption of both the inhalation and the exhalation

Overall, the *viloma pranayama* practice delivers most of the benefits we receive from other breath retention practices; however, each variation has its own unique benefits due to which part of the breath cycle is being interrupted and the associated effects on the autonomic nervous system.

VILOMA 1

Viloma 1 pauses the inhalation and has an uninterrupted exhalation. Of the three variations, it is the easiest for most people. The retentions follow the three parts of *dirgha svasam* (see pages 104 to 107), with the first retention after expanding the belly, the second after expanding the middle chest, and the third after filling the upper chest area. We can use a variety of techniques to apply the pauses. With all the *viloma* techniques, the breath cycle starts and finishes with a full end-expiratory volume exhalation, and each breath should be a complete vital capacity respiration. In other words, we should aim to fill the lungs to full capacity through our three-part breath and empty them as much as possible using a forced exhalation.

In *viloma* 1, the length of each of the three parts of the inhalation is intuitive, and the duration of each retention is also intuitive. The exhalation can be passive or slowed down. The other method is to use a ratio breathing pattern. The most common ratio taught with *viloma pranayama* is 1:2, with the first number representing the inhalation and the second number denoting the retention. For example, if you use a base of three, you would partially inhale to expand the belly for three seconds, hold for six seconds, partially inhale again for three seconds to fill the middle chest, hold again for six seconds, and then fully inhale for three more seconds to fill the upper chest, with a final hold of six seconds, followed by a complete exhalation. With this technique, I find it harder to hold the breath after the first inhalation and challenging to inhale for the final three seconds into the upper chest. I also find the last retention too short compared to my full inhalation.

My preferred method, and the way I teach my students, is based on a sliding ratio. It's a little more complicated but much more effective once you get used to practicing it. The first ratio is 3:2 to expand the belly. The second ratio is 2:3 to expand the middle chest, and the last ratio is 1:4 to expand the upper chest. With the sliding ratio, the longest inhalation with the shortest retention comes first, to expand the belly, and the shortest inhalation last, to fill the upper chest. The most prolonged retention is also when you have the most air in your lungs. The exhalation is a five-count, or a count equal to the combined length of the inhalation and retention. The full ratio is written like this:

3:2, 2:3, 1:4:5

VILOMA 1—3:2, 2:3, 1:4:5

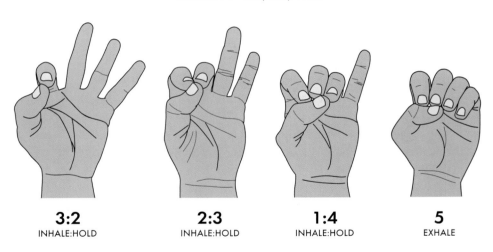

3:2	**2:3**	**1:4**	**5**
INHALE:HOLD	INHALE:HOLD	INHALE:HOLD	EXHALE

With the sliding ratio, I generally don't change these numbers like I would when practicing other breath ratios; instead, I slow the individual count. So counting to three could take three seconds, or it could take much longer. I aim to keep the speed of my count consistent throughout the practice. Just slowing the count makes it much easier to follow and allows a little influence from intuition. There is also a way to count on your fingers, which makes it simple to follow the ratio. If you start with an OK sign, three fingers up and the tips of the thumb and index finger joined, you have the first ratio of 3:2.

The fingers up are the inhalation, and the thumb and index finger are the retention. After the first part of the breath, lower the middle finger for the 2:3 ratio. For the last part of the breath, lower the index finger so that only the pinky is up, representing the inhalation, and the other four digits expressing the hold. Close the hand into a fist for the five-count exhalation. Return to the OK sign and start again.

If you don't like this method and want to be more exact with the count, you can change the numbers in the sliding ratio. For example, using a base of two seconds, the ratios would be 6:4, 4:6, 2:8:10, or, with a base of three seconds, the ratios would be 9:6, 6:9, 3:12:15.

Viloma 1 places the attention on the inhalation, which means it is slightly more energizing than the other two variations. Emphasizing the inhalation creates more *rajas* energy and more stimulation of the sympathetic nervous system. Because this is a retention practice, the parasympathetic nervous system is still dominant; however, *viloma* 1 is the most energizing of the three practices. When *viloma* 1 is combined with other energizing breaths, the energizing effects are much more apparent. *Viloma* 1 is a vital capacity breath, meaning each breath exercises the lower limit of the exhalation and the upper limit of the inhalation. The third step of the inhalation stretches the upper inspiratory muscles and increases vital capacity.

VILOMA 2

Viloma 2 is a smooth, continuous, full inhalation followed by retention interruptions on the exhalation. Like *viloma* 1, the pauses follow the three breath components of *dirgha svasam*. *Viloma* 2 has four breath retentions, adding *bahya kumbhaka* to the completion of the exhalation. The techniques are similar for all three *viloma pranayamas*. With the intuition method, the time it takes to inhale, exhale, and the length of the holds are intuitive. Start by taking a full exhalation, then slowly fill your lungs and hold *antara kumbhaka*. Exhale, contract your upper chest, hold the breath, exhale, contract your middle chest, hold the breath, exhale until completion, contract your stomach, and hold *bahya kumbhaka*. *Viloma* 2 still uses the 1:2 ratio, but here, the first number represents the exhalation; the second number remains the retention. I find the final retention much harder and longer compared to the rest of the retention in the exhalation.

With the sliding ratio method, you start with full exhalation followed by a five-count inhalation and five-count inner retention. The sliding ratio goes in reverse from *viloma* 1, starting with 1:4 (an exhalation of one and a retention of four). In the beginning, the exhalations are shortest and the retentions are longest. As you progress through the breath, the exhalations become the longest and the retentions become the shortest. The second ratio is 2:3, and the third ratio is 3:2. The ratio is written like this:

Inhalation 5:5 – Exhalation 1:4, 2:3, 3:2

VILOMA 2—Inhalation 5:5 – Exhalation 1:4, 2:3, 3:2

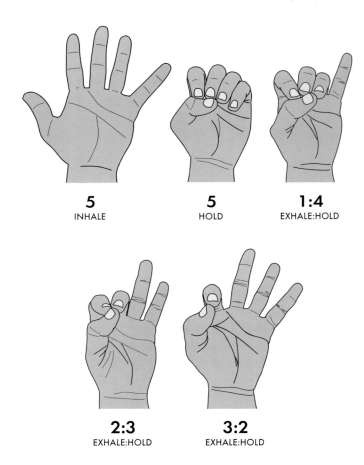

5
INHALE

5
HOLD

1:4
EXHALE:HOLD

2:3
EXHALE:HOLD

3:2
EXHALE:HOLD

To do this breath counting on the fingers, start with five fingers extended, representing the inhalation, followed by a fist for a five-count hold. Then lift your pinky, exhale for one count, and hold your breath for a four-count (one finger up, four fingers down). Lift your ring finger, exhale for a two-count, and hold the breath for a three-count. Lift your middle finger, making the "OK" sign, fully exhale for a three-count, and hold the breath for a two-count. Open

With *sitali* and *sitkari* breath, we lose all the advantages of breathing through the nose, like warming, humidifying, and filtering the incoming air. Therefore, doing these practices in a cold environment or when ill is not advised. Since the practice is done with an open mouth, there is less restriction when inhaling, so we can modify *sitali* if we want to inhale faster. Using this technique to breathe faster diminishes all the calming effects that we would typically see from the practice. However, it can be a great tool for cooling the body while increasing our energy levels and stimulating the sympathetic nervous system.

Sitali can also be paired with *simhasana pranayama,* or lion's breath, which is a wide-open-mouth exhale where we stick out our tongue and make a "ha" sound. The combination of the *sitali* inhalation with the *simhasana* exhalation exercises and stretches the muscles in the face and tongue and can be an effective energizing practice.

STEPS TO PRACTICE *SITALI PRANAYAMA*	
1	Start in a comfortable seated or kneeling position.
2	Open your mouth and make an "O" shape with your lips.
3	Stick out your tongue and curl up the sides. *
4	Engage *jalandhara bandha* (see pages 102 and 103).
5	Slowly inhale through the mouth. Use a breath ratio of 1:2.
6	Release *jalandhara bandha* and close your mouth.
7	Slowly exhale through the nose.
8	Repeat for 5 to 10 minutes.

*If you can't curl your tongue, press your teeth together and inhale through the teeth *(sitkari pranayama).*

SITALI PRANAYAMA EFFECTS
Cools the body
Promotes *tamas guna* (calm, cool, relaxed)

FIRE ESSENCE BREATH—*AGNISAR PRANAYAMA*

Agnisar pranayama, also known as *agnisar kriya,* is one of the ancient yogic cleansing techniques collectively called the *shat kriyas,* or "six actions." In Ayurveda (an ancient holistic system for natural healing that originated in India), *agnisar* is used to massage the visceral organs, eliminate toxins, help digestion, and boost metabolism. *Agni* means "fire," and *sar* means "essence." *Agnisar pranayama* shares many similarities and benefits with *bahya kumbhaka, uddiyana bandha* (see page 101), and *kapalabhati pranayama* (see pages 122 to 125).

You practice this breath while holding outer retention and then suck your stomach in and up, using the same technique as *uddiyana bandha.* While maintaining *bahya kumbhaka,* you pump your stomach in and out, similar to the action of *kapalabhati.* However, you do not inhale when releasing your stomach. The motion of the stomach pumping in and out increases blood flow to the abdominal organs and stimulates peristalsis: wavelike smooth muscle contractions in the intestines that aid in gut motility, digestion, and elimination. The practice increases the strength and endurance of the abdominal muscles, especially the deeper core muscles, accessory breathing muscles, and diaphragm. Studies have shown that strengthening the respiratory muscles and diaphragm improves respiratory function and boosts our resting metabolic rate.[7] Since the practice is done while holding the outer retention, it quickly builds up carbon dioxide levels in the body while making less air available in the lungs for gas exchange. As discussed in Section 1, having less available oxygen and more carbon dioxide stimulates the body to produce more red blood cells, which significantly increases athletic performance and VO_2 max.

Agnisar is a unique energetic practice; like *bhastrika* and *kapalabhati,* it is centered on the third *chakra* and is a powerful energy-increasing exercise. While it stimulates and supports the *rajas guna,* it is a *kumbhaka* practice, so there is an increase of carbon dioxide and stimulation of the parasympathetic nervous system. Whether you experience a calming effect or an energetic effect will come from the intention you have for your practice and the other breathing exercises you pair with *agnisar pranayama.*

When learning how to practice *agnisar kriya,* it can be helpful to start standing with your knees bent, hip width apart, and your hands on your knees in a tripod position. Or start in a seated or kneeling position, leaning forward with your hands braced on your knees. It's optional, but I also find it helpful to take ten to fifteen deep, fast breaths to create a mild carbon dioxide deficiency before holding the outer retention. The hypocapnia makes it much easier to hold the breath longer.

After the fast breathing, forcefully exhale as much air as possible out your mouth or nose. Hold the breath on the outer retention, tuck your chin to your chest, and engage *jalandhara bandha* (see pages 102 and 103). Contract your stomach by pulling your navel toward your spine as though you are trying to hollow out your belly by sucking in without actually inhaling. While still holding the breath, release and expand your abdomen by completely relaxing your core muscles. Repeat the pumping action of sucking in and contracting your belly and then releasing it.

In the beginning, aim for eight to ten repetitions per exhalation while focusing on making the action of contracting and releasing your stomach as smooth as possible. Take a slow, deep inhalation through the nose and repeat, starting with the ten to fifteen quick, deep breaths. Repeat for three to five rounds. Start slowly; as you build strength and coordination in your core, you can pump your belly faster. With practice, you'll be able to hold the *bahya kumbhaka* much longer, eventually getting thirty or more repetitions per breath.

AGINISAR

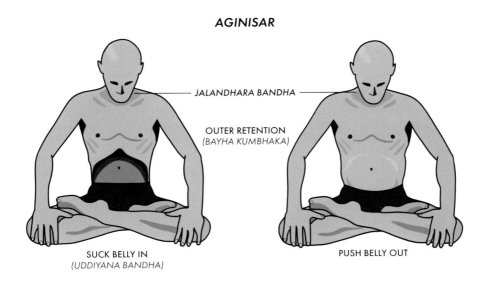

JALANDHARA BANDHA

OUTER RETENTION
(BAYHA KUMBHAKA)

SUCK BELLY IN
(UDDIYANA BANDHA)

PUSH BELLY OUT

Note: Practicing *agnisar pranayama* is not recommended if you are pregnant or you have gastrointestinal issues. *Agnisar* should be done on an empty stomach, preferably in the morning after a bowel movement.

STEPS TO PRACTICE *AGNISAR PRANAYAMA*

1	Start with your hands braced on your knees, either standing with your knees bent, hip width apart, or in a seated or kneeling position.
2	Take 10 to 15 fast, deep breaths.
3	Exhale completely and hold the breath.
4	Engage *jalandhara bandha* (see pages 102 and 103).
5	Rapidly pump your belly in and out as many times as possible while holding the breath.
6	Slowly inhale through the nose.
7	Repeat for 3 to 5 rounds.

AGNISAR PRANAYAMA EFFECTS

Aids in digestion and elimination (stimulates peristalsis, increases blood flow to the visceral organs)

Strengthens and tones abdominal muscles, increases endurance

Strengthens the diaphragm and other respiratory muscles

Increases athletic performance and VO_2 max (increases red blood cell production)

Boosts resting metabolic rate

Increases *rajas guna* (more energy, focus, productivity)

Stimulates the parasympathetic nervous system (rest and digest, calming effect)

NOTES

[1]Eva Bianconi et al., "An estimation of the number of cells in the human body," *Annals of Human Biology* 40, no. 6 (2013): 463–71, doi: 10.3109/03014460.2013.807878.

[2]Junjie Qin et al., "A human gut microbial gene catalogue established by metagenomic sequencing," *Nature* 464 (2010): 59–65, doi: 10.1038/nature08821.

[3]B. K. S. Iyengar, *Hatha Yoga Pradipika*, Yoga Swami Svatmarama. Unknown. Kindle Edition.

[4]I. M. Lin, L. Y. Tai, and S. Y. Fan, "Breathing at a rate of 5.5 breaths per minute with equal inhalation-to-exhalation ratio increases heart rate variability," *International Journal of Psychophysiology* 91, no. 3 (2014): 206–11, doi: 10.1016/j.ijpsycho.2013.12.006.

[5]Eddie Weitzberg and Jon O. N. Lundberg, "Humming greatly increases nasal nitric oxide," *American Journal of Respiratory and Critical Care Medicine* 166, no. 2 (2002): 144–5, doi: 10.1164/rccm.200202-138BC.

[6]R. Schulz, D. Schmidt, A. Blum, X. Lopes-Ribeiro, C. Lücke, K Mayer, H. Olschewski, W. Seeger, and F. Grimminger, "Decreased plasma levels of nitric oxide derivatives in obstructive sleep apnoea: response to CPAP therapy," *Thorax* 55 (2000): 1046–51, doi: 10.1136/thorax.55.12.1046.

[7]Min-Sik Yong, Yun-Seob Lee, and Hae-Yong Lee, "Effects of breathing exercises on resting metabolic rate and maximal oxygen uptake," *Journal of Physical Therapy Science* 30, no. 9 (2018): 1173–5, doi:10.1589/jpts.30.1173.

BREATH PRACTICE	ENERGETIC LEVEL	CARBON DIOXIDE	NITRIC OXIDE
UNEQUAL RATIO BREATHING *VISHAMA VRITTI*	SIGNIFICANTLY CALMING	SIGNIFICANT INCREASE	MILD INCREASE
HUMMING BEE BREATH *BHRAMARI*	MODERATELY CALMING	MILD INCREASE	SIGNIFICANT INCREASE
INTERRUPTED BREATHING 2 *VILOMA 2*	MILDLY CALMING	MODERATE INCREASE	MILD INCREASE
COOLING BREATH *SITALI/SITKARI*	MILDLY CALMING	MILD INCREASE	MODERATE DECREASE
INTERRUPTED BREATHING 3 *VILOMA 3*	BALANCING	MILD INCREASE	MILD INCREASE
THREE-PART BREATHING *DIRGHA SVASAM*	BALANCING	MILD INCREASE	MILD INCREASE
ALTERNATE NOSTRIL BREATHING *NADI SHODHANA*	BALANCING	MILD INCREASE	MILD INCREASE
EQUAL RATIO BREATHING *SAMA VRITTI*	BALANCING	MODERATE INCREASE	MILD INCREASE
INTERRUPTED BREATHING 1 *VILOMA 1*	MILDLY ENERGIZING	MILD INCREASE	MILD INCREASE
VICTORIOUS BREATH *UJJAYI*	MILDLY ENERGIZING	MILD DECREASE	MILD INCREASE
BREATH OF FIRE *AGNI PRAN*	MODERATELY ENERGIZING	MODERATE DECREASE	MILD DECREASE
SKULL SHINING BREATH *KAPALABHATI*	SIGNIFICANTLY ENERGIZING	SIGNIFICANT DECREASE	MILD DECREASE
BELLOWS BREATH *BHASTRIKA*	SIGNIFICANTLY ENERGIZING	SIGNIFICANT DECREASE	MILD DECREASE
FIRE ESSENCE BREATH *AGNISAR*	SIGNIFICANTLY ENERGIZING	SIGNIFICANT INCREASE	MILD DECREASE

PHYSIOLOGICAL EFFECTS

NERVOUS SYSTEM	GUNA	NADI	VAYU
PARASYMPATHETIC/ DORSAL VAGAL COMPLEX	TAMAS	IDA	SAMANA
PARASYMPATHETIC/ DORSAL VAGAL COMPLEX	TAMAS	IDA	UDANA
PARASYMPATHETIC/ DORSAL VAGAL COMPLEX	TAMAS	IDA	APANA
PARASYMPATHETIC/ DORSAL VAGAL COMPLEX	TAMAS	IDA	VYANA
PARASYMPATHETIC/ VENTRAL VAGAL COMPLEX	SATTVA	SUSHUMNA	PRANA
PARASYMPATHETIC/ VENTRAL VAGAL COMPLEX	SATTVA	SUSHUMNA	PRANA
PARASYMPATHETIC/ VENTRAL VAGAL COMPLEX	SATTVA	SUSHUMNA	PRANA
PARASYMPATHETIC/ VENTRAL VAGAL COMPLEX	SATTVA	SUSHUMNA	PRANA
SYMPATHETIC	SATTVA/RAJAS	PINGALA	UDANA
SYMPATHETIC	RAJAS	PINGALA	VYANA
SYMPATHETIC	RAJAS	PINGALA	UDANA
SYMPATHETIC	RAJAS	PINGALA	UDANA
SYMPATHETIC	RAJAS	PINGALA	VYANA
PARASYMPATHETIC/ DORSAL VAGAL COMPLEX	RAJAS	PINGALA	SAMANA

SYSTEMS OF BALANCE

STANDARD EFFECTS FROM *PRANAYAMA* PRACTICES. MODIFYING PRACTICES, COMBINING EXERCISES, OR CHANGING BREATHING SPEEDS WILL CHANGE THE PHYSIOLOGICAL AND ENERGETIC EFFECTS.

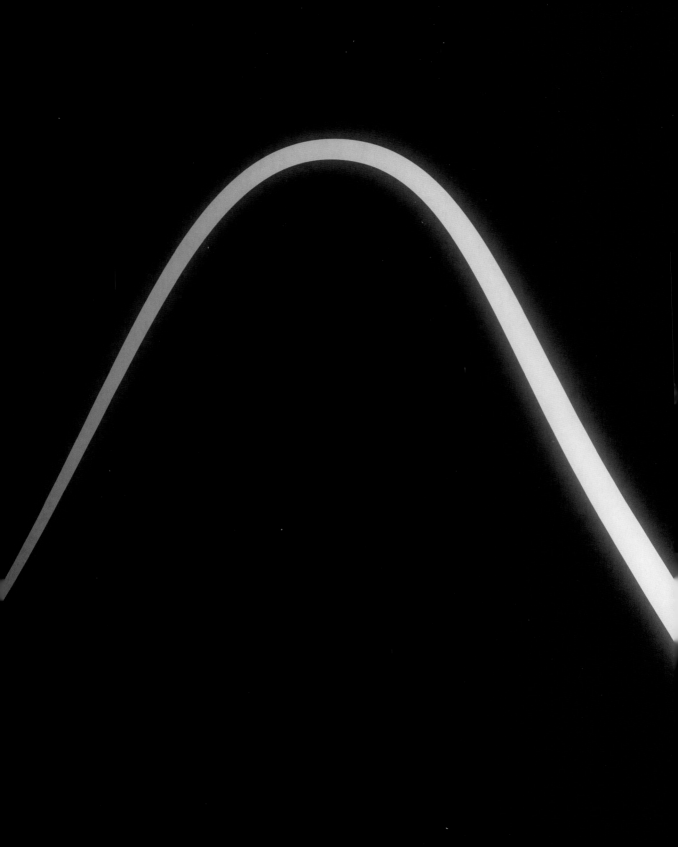

[SECTION 4]
CREATING A BREATH SEQUENCE

As we've discussed in great detail, the breath is a powerful tool that we can use to influence everything from our health to our happiness. Every breathing technique we learn is like another tool added to our toolbox, with most of these tools being multipurpose. But, like most multifunctional tools, they are never as good as a device that was specifically designed for a singular purpose. If you're an artist, for example, you might have an array of brushes that you use to achieve specific effects. If you're a poet or a writer, the meanings of the words that you use can vary dramatically depending on the context in which you use them. And if you're a storyteller, how you structure the plot and develop the characters can captivate the listener and take them on an emotional ride that immerses them in the story.

Creating a breath practice to effect positive change and influence our health and well-being is not much different. A breathing technique that has a plethora of uses can be modified and improved for a more precise application. For example, the victorious breath *(ujjayi pranayama)* increases energy and stimulates sympathetic tone through increased respirations and deeper breathing. The technique used to create the *ujjayi* sound can also stimulate parasympathetic tone by increasing pressure on the vagus nerve. By modifying the *ujjayi* technique, we can get more of what we want and less of what we don't. So, we customize each technique by changing the lengths of the inhalations and exhalations or the durations of the breath-holds. We can combine two or three *pranayama* practices, pulling specific elements from each one to create a new breathing exercise that physically or energetically brings us closer to our goal or intention. We can also sequence multiple techniques to give context to the breath and accentuate the effects of each method.

Pranayama and even Western breathing exercises, such as the 4-7-8 breath (see page 120) and the recovery breath, are usually practiced unaccompanied by other breathing exercises. Doing a singular exercise can be like painting with a broad brush: it covers a lot of area but doesn't get the fine detail that we need to create a compelling work of art. Sometimes I see two or three *pranayama* techniques practiced together, but the combination doesn't move toward a specific goal. Why we are doing these particular exercises together is often not understood; usually, there wasn't an overlying intention for the practice to begin with.

A breath practice without cohesion is like a yoga class in which the teacher calls out a series of random poses that have no relationship or flow. We might receive a small benefit, but because the class is all over the place, we won't get as much out of it as we would have if the class had targeted a specific intention or purpose. Doing any conscious breathing, whether it is a single exercise or a combination of techniques, will have positive effects. However, when we have a set intention and choose specific methods to accomplish that purpose, the benefits we receive will be so much more significant.

BREATH SEQUENCE CONSIDERATIONS

There are a few things to consider when doing a breath practice or teaching a breath practice to others:

- What is our goal or intention?

- Which *pranayama* or other breathing exercises work toward that goal or intention?

- How can we change or modify those breathing techniques to better fit our intention for the breath?

- How can we pair a breathing exercise with another exercise to accentuate the desired effect of each technique?

- How can we sequence the different techniques to create a cohesive practice that energetically moves in a way that is conducive to our goal or intention?

- How long should the breath practice be?

Let's look at each of these questions individually.

WHAT IS OUR GOAL OR INTENTION?

Goal and intention might seem like they are the same thing. Often they feel similar and even overlap, but we should view them differently. The *goal* is what we are trying to achieve or are working toward with the practice. The *intention* is about why we are working toward that goal.

When setting the goal, it's essential to consider the intention behind that goal. Often, the intention helps us choose the right breathing exercises to accomplish our goal. For example, if your goal was to hold your breath longer, you would ask yourself, "*Why* do I want to hold my breath longer?" The benefits of holding the breath range from increasing athletic performance and VO_2 max to lowering blood pressure and heart rate to calming the mind for meditation. The way to approach breath retention for increasing athletic performance is very different from the method with which we practice holding the breath to prepare the mind for meditation. What if the goal is not about holding the breath longer, but *is* meditation? Then you can refine your intention to clarify why you want to meditate. Do you want to meditate to feel more equanimous as you prepare for your day, or do you want to meditate on moving into deep relaxation as you end your day?

The process of defining a goal and understanding the intention behind it should lead us to a place where the goal and the intention are in perfect harmony. Arriving at this point will make it easy to choose and modify the breathing techniques for the practice.

WHICH *PRANAYAMA* OR OTHER BREATHING EXERCISES WILL WORK TOWARD OUR GOAL OR INTENTION?

It's important to have a decent understanding of the different *pranayama* techniques outlined in Section 3 and how they affect the mind and body—not only to understand them intellectually but to have experienced them through hours of practice. When we are trying to pick the best breathing practices to support the achievement of a goal, we are searching first for broad-stroke brushes that we can refine later.

When choosing the techniques for each practice, we want to consider the following:

- The energetic effects
- The emotional or spiritual effects
- The physical effects

The energetic effects will increase energy, decrease energy, or create balance generally based on how it affects our autonomic nervous system and the other systems of balance. If the goal of the breath sequence is to be more alert in the morning, then we want to choose more energizing practices. Conversely, if it is to help with deep sleep, then we want more calming practices. For the most part, practices with faster respirations have an energizing effect, such as *bhastrika* or *kapalabhati.* Slower respirations and holds have a calming effect, such as *vishama vritti* or any *kumbhaka* practice, and more equal ratio breathing practices have an energetic balancing effect, like *sama vritti* or *dirgha svasam.*

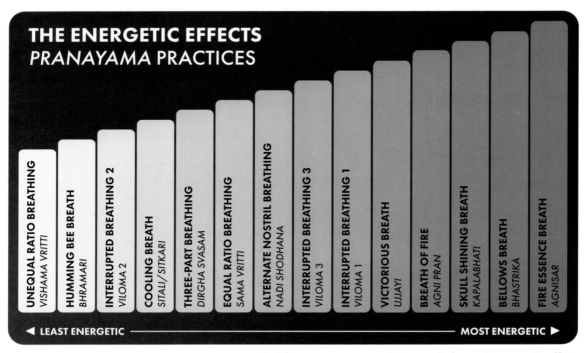

Modifying a *pranayama* technique will change its energetic effect.

Finding the right practice to help with an emotional or spiritual goal can be challenging and requires a little more understanding of the *nadis* (see page 65), *gunas* (see page 70), and *prana vayus* (see page 77). Also, when the goal is emotional or spiritual, setting a strong intention can have more of an impact than the chosen *pranayama* practice. The practice then becomes secondary to energetically support the intention. Each Eastern system of balance can be used as a map to guide us in support of the intention. Consult the graphs and descriptions in the book to find the *nadi, guna,* or *prana vayu* that best represents your emotional or spiritual goal, then find the corresponding breathing practice on the *pranayama* effects chart (see pages 154 and 155).

For example, if the goal is equanimity, we can use a practice that promotes the *sushumna nadi,* such as *nadi shodhana.* If the intention is about compassion, we can look to *sattva guna* and use *sama vritti* for the breathing practice. For an intention such as creating more intimacy, we would want to focus on *apana vayu,* and we can choose *viloma* 2 to help support the intention.

PRANAYAMA PRACTICES FOR THE *NADIS*

BELLOWS BREATH
BHASTRIKA

SKULL SHINING BREATH
KAPALABHATI

BREATH OF FIRE
AGNI PRAN

VICTORIOUS BREATH
UJJAYI

FIRE ESSENCE BREATH
AGNISAR

INTERRUPTED BREATHING 1
VILOMA 1

INTERRUPTED BREATHING 3
VILOMA 3

ALTERNATE NOSTRIL BREATHING
NADI SHODHANA

EQUAL RATIO BREATHING
SAMA VRITTI

THREE-PART BREATHING
DIRGHA SVASAM

UNEQUAL RATIO BREATHING
VISHAMA VRITTI

HUMMING BEE BREATH
BHRAMARI

COOLING BREATH
SITALI / SITKARI

INTERRUPTED BREATHING 2
VILOMA 2

PINGALA   **SUSHUMNA**   **IDA**

UDANA

HUMMING BEE BREATH
BHRAMARI

SKULL SHINING BREATH
KAPALABHATI

INTERRUPTED BREATHING 1
VILOMA 1

BREATH OF FIRE
AGNI PRAN

VYANA

VICTORIOUS BREATH
UJJAYI

BELLOWS BREATH
BHASTRIKA

COOLING BREATH
SITALI/SITKARI

PRANA

THREE-PART BREATHING
DIRGHA SVASAM

EQUAL RATIO BREATHING
SAMA VRITTI

ALTERNATE NOSTRIL BREATHING
NADI SHODHANA

INTERRUPTED BREATHING 3
VILOMA 3

SAMANA

FIRE ESSENCE BREATH
AGNISAR

UNEQUAL RATIO BREATHING
VISHAMA VRITTI

APANA

INTERRUPTED BREATHING 2
VILOMA 2

When determining which breathing exercises move toward achieving a physical or health-related goal, we generally start by asking a few questions relating to our desired physiological outcome.

- Is the trait affected by either increased or decreased levels of carbon dioxide and blood pH?

- Does this attribute receive a benefit from increasing nitric oxide levels?

- How does the state of our autonomic nervous system affect the physical outcome relating to our goal?

You can use the charts "The Effects of Hyperventilation vs. Hypoventilation" (see page 35) and "The Autonomic Nervous System" (see page 53) or revisit the effects of nitric oxide (see pages 24 to 26) to choose the exercises that will help achieve the goal. The better your understanding of the physiological effects of breathing and the nervous system, the easier this task will be. For example, if the goal is to lower blood pressure, then we would look for practices that increase carbon dioxide since we know that higher carbon dioxide levels decrease blood pressure. Any type of *kumbhaka* practice is going to be effective. For certain intentions, we might need to refine some of our questions or search outside the box. For example, if the goal is to run faster, we want to think about the things that boost our athletic performance, such as increasing VO_2 max and lung capacity. For VO_2 max, we want exercises that lower our SpO_2 to make more oxygen-carrying red blood cells, such as *bahya kumbhaka* or *viloma* 2. And for lung capacity, we know that *viloma* 1 and *dirgha svasam* are great practices.

THE PHYSICAL EFFECTS
PRANAYAMA PRACTICES

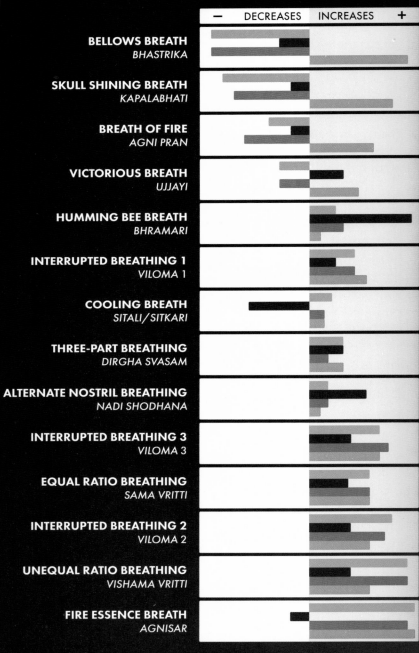

CARBON DIOXIDE
NITRIC OXIDE
VO$_2$ MAX
STRENGTH*

*Respiratory muscle strength

— DECREASES   INCREASES +

BELLOWS BREATH
BHASTRIKA

SKULL SHINING BREATH
KAPALABHATI

BREATH OF FIRE
AGNI PRAN

VICTORIOUS BREATH
UJJAYI

HUMMING BEE BREATH
BHRAMARI

INTERRUPTED BREATHING 1
VILOMA 1

COOLING BREATH
SITALI/SITKARI

THREE-PART BREATHING
DIRGHA SVASAM

ALTERNATE NOSTRIL BREATHING
NADI SHODHANA

INTERRUPTED BREATHING 3
VILOMA 3

EQUAL RATIO BREATHING
SAMA VRITTI

INTERRUPTED BREATHING 2
VILOMA 2

UNEQUAL RATIO BREATHING
VISHAMA VRITTI

FIRE ESSENCE BREATH
AGNISAR

Modifying a *pranayama* practice will change its physical effects.

HOW CAN WE CHANGE OR MODIFY A BREATHING TECHNIQUE TO BETTER FIT OUR GOAL OR INTENTION?

We experience several effects from every breathing technique. Each breath practice has either an emotional impact (the influence of our energetic body, such as the *gunas, vayus,* and *nadis*) or a physiological effect (how the breath influences the autonomic nervous system, stimulating either the sympathetic nervous system, the dorsal vagal complex, or the ventral vagal complex). Both the science-based Western approach of the autonomic nervous system and the polyvagal theory and the Eastern philosophical yogic view of the subtle energy body are essentially maps of our emotions, spirit, and vigor. The two systems work together, like different languages describing the same things. For example:

- The sympathetic nervous system, *rajas guna, pingala nadi, udana vayu,* and *vyana vayu* all relate to how energy increases or expands.

- The dorsal vagal complex, *tamas guna, ida nadi, apana vayu,* and *samana vayu* all express how energy decreases or contracts.

- The ventral vagal complex, *sattva guna, sushumna nadi,* and *prana vayu* all describe balance and harmony.

Each map points out certain nuances. When we know the goal and intention, we can choose whether it makes sense to focus on practices that emphasize one system or whether it is better to draw from all the energetic systems. This high level of detail is not critical but can help us pick the right practices for our carefully thought out intention. If in doubt, choose practices that move toward the overall energetic goal—i.e., increasing or expanding energy, decreasing or contracting energy, or balancing energy.

The breath practices also affect our physiology by changing our blood chemistry and influencing our autonomic nervous system. We can use our knowledge of how speeding up or slowing down the breath or adding retention changes blood pH and carbon dioxide levels to modify every breath practice to better suit our intention. We can also combine breathing exercises that have other physiological effects, like increasing nitric oxide to amplify or suppress the effects of other breath practices, to enhance our intended results.

As much of an influence as the autonomic nervous system has on our emotional and energetic body, it has an equal influence on the cardiac, respiratory, metabolic, digestive, and other biological systems. If I am trying to understand emotions and feelings, the polyvagal theory explains this better. However, when we look at how the autonomic nervous system affects our physiology, the traditional two-branch sympathetic and parasympathetic nervous system theory is much more useful and easier to follow:

- Speeding up the breath or lengthening the inhalation affects the sympathetic nervous system.

- Slowing down the breath or extending the exhalation affects the parasympathetic nervous system.

Using these simple methods, we can modify a breath practice to alter our blood pressure, heart rate, digestion, or other biological functions. Sometimes our intention will require us to look at both theories of the autonomic nervous system to find or modify the breathing practice(s) that will help us accomplish our goal.

After choosing a breathing technique, we evaluate all the effects of that practice that move us toward our goal or intention. Then we see if we can change things like the rate of breathing or the breath ratio to help us achieve our goal. For example, if we want a practice that is emotionally balancing yet physically energizing, we can speed up the respirations for *nadi shodhana.* Or, if we have two exercises that are synergistic, like *nadi shodhana* and box breathing (both balancing practices), we may want to combine them to create a new exercise.

Along with the desired results, a breath practice often has other outcomes that could be counterproductive to our goal and intention. Sometimes modifying the practice diminishes the unwanted side effects, and sometimes we need to alter the practice to attain the effects we want. For example, if we are trying to increase our energy with *bhastrika pranayama* but we don't want the adverse effects that come with hyperventilation, we can use a breath retention practice to increase our carbon dioxide levels. If the changes still leave us with undesired effects, we might want to opt for another technique or sequence the breath practice with other breathing exercises that help highlight our overall intention. In other words, multiple modifications are available, and every practice can be adapted to serve our needs. Finally, we can determine if we can integrate any other breathing practices or components of a technique to improve the energetic or physiological effect of the sequence.

HOW CAN WE PAIR A BREATHING EXERCISE WITH ANOTHER EXERCISE TO ACCENTUATE THE DESIRED EFFECT OF EACH TECHNIQUE?

So much of our understanding of life comes from context. Whether it's a situation, a word, or, in this case, a breathing exercise, the framework in which we experience a thing gives it as much, if not more, meaning than the thing itself. We experience this every day as we communicate. A word in one sentence might have a completely different meaning than the same word in another sentence. For example, we all can agree that *love* means something different when I say, "I love my mother" versus "I love my partner" versus "I love burritos." The three statements share the connotation of having an affinity toward something. However, your love for your partner is considerably different from your love for burritos. At least I hope it is!

Sometimes context can change a word's meaning or even its pronunciation. Take the word *tear:* "I tear the paper" versus "I cried a single tear." Because of context, we can take a breathing practice like *kumbhaka* and, without modifying it, combine it with other exercises that will help increase athletic performance or promote a state of deep relaxation.

In yoga, for example, a good teacher will create a sequence of poses that move the class toward a specific goal or intention, such as opening the hips, back-bending, or doing forward folds. Or the teacher might have an energetic intention and choose poses that express the qualities of that energy. Many postures have multiple purposes. For example, *camatkarasana,* the posture better known as "wild thing," influences several physical benefits, such as opening the hips and psoas, deepening backbends, stretching the sides of the body, and strengthening the arms and legs. It does all these things and more, but it doesn't do any of them that well. For every benefit of wild thing, there is another pose that does it better. However, when *camatkarasana* is used in the context of a back-bending or hip-opening class, it adds variety and interest to the other movements, and the purpose of including this pose becomes more apparent. A student feels the intention of the class through that pose. A skilled yoga teacher can take a standard pose like wild thing and modify it slightly to make it work even better for the overall intention of the class.

Bhramari pranayama is amazing for increasing nitric oxide, and because of the wide array of effects that nitric oxide has, we must choose other breathing practices to highlight the effects we want. For example, if we combine *bhramari* with *nadi shodhana,* the calming and balancing aspects of *nadi shodhana* will enhance the relaxing effects created by the increased nitric oxide. If we add *bhramari* to the energizing and lower *chakra*–stimulating *agni sar* practice, we can showcase how nitric oxide increases libido.

Adding context to a breathing exercise by placing it with other similar and synergistic breathing exercises creates meaning that defines the intention. The exercises in a sequence should have variety and portray different parts of the story that lead to the same conclusion.

HOW CAN WE LINK VARIOUS BREATHING TECHNIQUES TO CREATE A COHESIVE PRACTICE THAT ENERGETICALLY MOVES TOWARD OUR GOAL OR INTENTION?

If you've ever worked out, gone running, or taken a yoga class, you probably started with some sort of warm-up, moved into the more physical part, and concluded with a cool-down and some stretches. Most people don't start with sprints or try to hit their personal record without adequate preparation. With fitness, most people follow some sort of energetic arc.

When I teach a yoga class, I structure the sequence using an energetic arc called a sequence wave, which includes an opening, a gentle warm-up, a heat-building component, a dynamic or vitalizing component, a cool-down, *savasana,* and a closing. I slowly build up the energy of the class, come to a crescendo in the sequence, and then bring the energy back down. A good sequence creates a narrative that pulses like a compelling story through every aspect of the class. The warm-up and heat-building sections foreshadow more difficult poses revealed in the dynamic component and then resolve in the cool-down. The way I create a breath sequence follows many of the same principles.

When creating a breath sequence, think of it as a story, where the essence of the narrative weaves a cohesive intention with every breathing exercise and *pranayama* technique. The overall intention of the sequence should be experienced in each individual exercise, leading us down a clear path to express our goal. The entirety of the sequence should feel like the rise and fall of a single deep breath that starts easy and then expands with intensity. The deeper the inhalation, the more challenge we experience until we reach the apex of inspiration and release it, to descend the exhalation, concluding with a harmonious resolution.

HOW LONG SHOULD THE BREATH PRACTICE BE?

Having a breath practice is similar to having a meditation practice, yoga practice, or fitness routine. There isn't a specific amount of time that we *should* practice breathing. It's best to start with a length that you feel comfortable with and build up from there. When I teach students how to practice meditation on their own, I encourage them to start by doing five minutes a day to build a habit. A mistake many people make when it comes to adding anything new into their lives is that they start with more than they can handle and quit before they can either establish a routine or experience the benefits in order to understand the value of the practice. Even though five minutes a day won't have much of an impact compared to thirty minutes or an hour, creating a daily habit is paramount. It's the same with fitness: working out every day for five minutes is better than working out once a month for two and a half hours. When we create a habit, it's easy to incrementally increase the time we dedicate to it without radically changing our daily routine. The more time we dedicate, the more benefits we receive, but the key is consistency.

Creating a short breath sequence is often difficult because each component of the sequence may contain multiple time-bound breathing exercises that are not practical to remove. Still, a ten-minute sequence can be manageable and sufficient for certain intentions. Emotional and energetic changes can be experienced relatively quickly; even with just a few breaths, we begin to feel a difference. Despite these quick energetic changes, most physical goals are difficult to achieve with a short breathing practice. Significant physiological change typically manifests after prolonged application. For example, we can immediately change our blood pH and affect our autonomic nervous system, but for longer-lasting results, we need to spend more time in the practice, especially if we center the practice on breath retention.

If all you have is five minutes, then doing a five-minute practice is better than not doing any practice at all. You quickly want to establish a ten- to fifteen-minute daily practice and then gradually increase to thirty minutes or longer a day. Once you maintain a thirty-minute daily breathing practice for a few months, you'll be an expert on how long or short you should make your practice to keep it effective.

Changing the duration of a breath sequence is simple. As detailed in the following section, breath sequences have four sections or components. Each component consists of one or more breathing exercises. To lengthen or shorten a sequence, we change the number of repetitions of each exercise. For example, if the first component includes one exercise consisting of five repetitions totaling two and a half minutes and we want to increase the duration to five minutes, we double the repetitions. In short, we can add or take away from each exercise until we arrive at the duration we want.

When choosing how long or how many repetitions for each breathing exercise, evaluate the duration you need to practice in order to feel the results. The best way to determine this is to practice each technique and determine when you start to notice physiological or energetic changes, such as feeling calmer or having more energy. With breath sequencing, we are working with two factors—the length of each individual section and the overall length of the sequence—and both need to be considered. Let your intention guide you. I find that mine usually leads me to the right place if I take time to listen.

THE BREATH SEQUENCE WAVE

The energetic arc that I use to sequence a breath practice is slightly different from the sequence wave that I use for my yoga classes, but it follows the same basic structure.

If we are teaching a breath sequence to other people, we start with an introduction or opening. When I teach a *pranayama* class, which follows the breath-sequencing principles laid out in this book, I begin by explaining the goal and intention of the breath sequence. I then list all the breathing exercises that we will do in the class. I briefly explain why I have chosen these specific techniques and then demonstrate how to do each one. To maintain the energetic wave and ensure that my students get the most benefit both physically and emotionally, I avoid disruptions to the flow of the practice. By explaining each technique before we start the sequence, I can cue and count the breath without having to stop and explain the next breathing exercise.

If we are not sharing our breath sequence with others, taking a moment to review our intention and memorizing the sequence will be just as helpful.

The breath sequence wave has four components that act as a guide and a tool to create a cohesive structure:

- Warm-up

- Heat-building

- Vitalizing

- Cool-down

I usually build a sequence by starting with the vitalizing section, followed by heat-building, and then I create the warm-up and cool-down centered around the bulk of the class that leads me toward my goal. You may find it more helpful to begin with another component, such as the warm-up, and move in chronological order. The sequence wave is designed to be a tool to organize the energetic arc. The order in which the sequence is created doesn't matter as long as it's practiced in the order listed above.

Depending on the goal, these four components might express themselves very differently. A heat-building breathing exercise for an energizing intention will be much different from a heat-building exercise for a relaxing intention.

Each component of the breath sequence can have one or more breathing exercises, or a component may be omitted from the sequence if its energetics don't fit the overall intention. For example, you might choose not to create a heat-building exercise for a deep relaxation breath sequence. The length of each component depends on the duration and difficulty of the entire sequence. Generally, more difficult or intense practices will have longer heat-building and vitalizing components. A more passive or subtle practice will place the focus on the warm-up and cool-down. If the duration of each section is similar, then the sequence will feel more balanced. We can see that the energy of the *gunas* is present even when it comes to the structure of the breath sequence. The breath sequence wave is another tool that we can use to push the intention of our practice and express the energetic amplitude that we want to convey.

Before beginning the first breathing exercise in a sequence, you want to check in with yourself, without judgment and without trying to immediately change your current condition. In other words, always begin at your baseline. If there is somewhere you need to go, the breath work will take you there. Begin by observing the quality of your breath, including the rate, rhythm, and depth. While you monitor the breath, you want to let it flow naturally. As you breathe, observe how you feel energetically. Do you feel low on energy, highly energized, or balanced? Also make a note of your emotional state. Notice if you are feeling calm and relaxed or if agitation, anxiety, or any other emotions arise as you sit with the breath. You should start every practice by observing the baseline of your physical and mental condition so that you have something to compare to how you are feeling at the end of the practice.

After establishing a baseline, take a few moments to center in and create a mind-body connection to your breath. You can easily form this connection by taking a few slow, conscious breaths in and out through the nose. Adding a few short breath-holds can also be helpful, especially if we are feeling anxious or agitated.

BREATH SEQUENCE WAVE

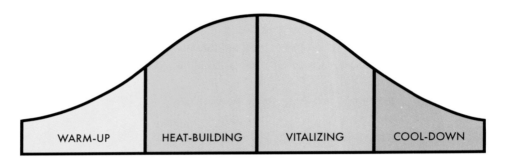

| WARM-UP | HEAT-BUILDING | VITALIZING | COOL-DOWN |

THE WARM-UP

If you are going for a run, you want to spend some time warming up your muscles. The same is true for breathing: you want to take adequate time to warm up the diaphragm and respiratory muscles.

Consider the energetic quality or *guna* that you wish to express. For example, if you are working with the *rajas guna* (increased energy), then the warm-up will be more intense compared to a sequence centered on the *tamas guna* (decreased energy). If the intention is *sattvic* (balancing energy), then the warm-up could be either a balanced, *sattvic* breathing exercise or one that is more *rajasic* that is later resolved with a *tamasic* breathing exercise in the cool-down.

It's important to note that *warm-up* doesn't mean *easy*. *Warm-up* is a relative term, like hot or cold. Water at 100°F (38°C) is cool compared to boiling water and hot compared to ice water. The intensity of the warm-up should reflect the energy of the breath sequence. If the sequence is challenging, then the warm-up should reflect the same difficulty. The primary purpose of the warm-up is to prepare the mind and body for the more rigorous exercises to come while establishing the intention for the sequence.

Developing a warm-up can be challenging if you don't know what you are warming up for. As mentioned earlier, this why I often create the vitalizing component first. Knowing what comes next allows us to foreshadow the rest of the sequence. Foreshadowing is when an exercise alludes to a practice(s) that will be done later in the sequence, either by creating a modification or variation of the future practice or doing a similar type or style of breathing exercise. For example, if the vitalizing component involves a long breath retention, then the warm-up should include a shorter retention. Foreshadowing isn't necessary, but it can be a great way to introduce an easier variation of a more complex practice that will be done later in the sequence, which enables us to prepare for the challenge. Foreshadowing also gives the practice an overall cohesion and emphasizes our intention. If we decide not to foreshadow with the warm-up, we should consider the type(s) of breathing exercises in the vitalizing and heat-building sections and choose warm-up techniques that build up to the later, more challenging exercises.

The warm-up can be

- A singular breathing exercise that is repeated throughout the section

- A slow ramping up of an exercise that starts easy and gradually becomes slightly more challenging

- A series of several breathing exercises that sequentially increase in intensity

THE HEAT-BUILDING COMPONENT

The primary function of the heat-building component is to amplify the intensity of the practice. Just like the warm-up, it needs to address the overall energetic quality of the sequence while considering the vitalizing component and the goal of the practice. In a breath sequence that has a calming or relaxed energy, the heat-building section will be very mild and seem more like an extension of the warm-up or a precursor to the vitalizing section.

There are several ways to increase the intensity of the practice. If the sequence focuses on *rajas guna,* then one option is to use a faster breathing exercise, such as *kapalabhati* or *bhastrika.* Any type of rapid breathing is going to stimulate the sympathetic nervous system, increase the heart rate and blood pressure, raise cardiorespiratory demand, and boost metabolism. These physiological changes build heat in the body and amplify mental energy and concentration. We can also use fast breathing techniques when the sequence centers on the *sattva guna;* however, we need to balance the rapid breathing with a breath retention practice. Some type of breath retention exercise will likely follow any practice that increases the respiratory rate. Both rapid breathing and breath retention can be a part of the heat-building section or a part of the same breathing exercise. We can also use a fast breathing exercise in the heat-building section to prepare for a challenging *kumbhaka* practice in the vitalizing section.

Most *pranayama* practices stimulate the cardiorespiratory system and therefore already function to build heat and intensity. How we approach or use a breath practice in the sequence will give it context as to whether it belongs in that section of the sequence. It is the context of the sequence that we use to find the appropriate breathing exercises for the heat-building section. Beyond building heat, this section is responsible for bridging the gap between the warm-up and the vitalizing section.

THE VITALIZING COMPONENT

The vitalizing or dynamic component is the crescendo of the practice. This section is where the intention or goal is fully realized and expressed. It is essentially the most important component because it gives the rest of the sequence its context.

When choosing the exercise(s) for the vitalizing component, we need to break down the goal of the sequence. Is there an emotional aspect to the goal? If we are trying to feel an expression of an emotion, then our primary concern is addressing this emotional aspect. Guiding emotions is incredibly challenging, but following the breath can be simple. Therefore, we need to be precise with our intention to follow the breath in a way that will create the emotional transformation we are seeking.

The *vayus* offer us a beautiful map to understand the movement of feelings and how to rebalance our emotions. The *vayus* address the imbalances of the movement of emotional energies and the stagnation that creates dysfunction and suffering. When we set a goal for an emotional change, we want to design the practice to bring us from the antithesis of that emotional goal. In other words, if we want a breath practice that makes us happy, we are creating a practice that assumes we are sad. But if the goal is something like being happy, then it would serve us to refine our understanding of the conditions of our unhappiness, or our energetic imbalance, because an emotion like unhappiness can have many causes. Once we define the source of the imbalance or the contrasting emotion of our goal emotion, we can find where that imbalance lies in the *vayus* and follow the breath to resolve that imbalance. Emotional practices are subtle and require a lot of intention to be effective. *Mudras* and visualization can be beneficial elements in aiding the purpose of the breath practice.

What is the desired physical outcome of our goal? Are we trying to effect a physiological change? The physical aspect may be the main component of the goal, like increasing athletic performance or improving memory. Or it can be a synergistic quality that supports our intention. For example, if the goal is to decrease stress and anxiety, we want a practice that helps lower our blood pressure and pulse. When we are choosing *pranayama* practices or other breathing techniques, we want to consider their effects on the autonomic nervous system and other physiological changes that come from the breath, like carbon dioxide and nitric oxide. Finding breathing exercises that affect us physically is much easier and more straightforward than it is for emotional goals.

What is the energetic quality of our goal: *rajas, tamas,* or *sattva*? The energetic aspect gives us insight into how we should be breathing. We know that if we want more energy, we breathe faster; for less energy, we breathe slower. It's important to remember that some breathing exercises paradoxically increase *rajasic* energy and parasympathetic tone. There are also practices that increase *tamasic* energy and sympathetic tone. But generally, the *rajas guna* follows the sympathetic nervous system and the *tamas guna* accompanies the parasympathetic nervous system.

THE COOL-DOWN

The cool-down expresses the resolution of the intention. Sometimes the cool-down echoes a softer variation of the vitalizing component or mirrors the warm-up, culminating the practice. Again, we need to consider the objective of the practice and the energetic quality associated with our goal. With most practices, the cool-down is one energetic step down from the intensity of the rest of the sequence. For example:

- If the energy of the sequence is *rajas,* then the cool-down will feel *sattvic.*

- If the energy is *sattva,* then the cool-down will feel *tamasic.*

- And if the energy is *tamas,* then the cool-down will remain at the same intensity.

This ramp-down in intensity (or sustaining of *tamas*) gives a conclusive feeling to the practice and gives the sequence an overall impression of balance and harmony.

If the intention for the sequence is emotional, then the cool-down should reflect that intention so that we are left feeling the intended sentiment. Again, accompanying the breath with *mudras* and visualization can be an excellent way to bring awareness to the emotional quality manifested by the intention.

If the practice has a physiological goal, the cool-down can serve to support or resolve that goal. When the entire sequence feels balanced, we choose milder practices for the cool-down that continue to effect the physical outcome represented in the rest of the sequence. If the sequence leading up to the cool-down pulls us too much in one direction or leaves us feeling out of balance, we resolve the goal with practices that counter the actions of the vitalizing section and restore balance. We usually only need to counter when the vitalizing section consists of breathing exercises that have too much sympathetic tone. Even when the goal of a breath sequence centers on increasing sympathetic tone, we want to conclude the practice with a more balanced autonomic nervous system so that we are able to return to the healthy resting breath. We never want our breath sequences to result in over-breathing or other long-term poor breathing habits.

THE CONCLUSION AND CHECK-IN

After concluding the breath sequence, we want to consciously breathe for a minimum of five to ten respirations to allow adequate time to return to the resting breath and reestablish good breathing habits. We should also take time to check in with how we are feeling post-practice. Just as we took the time to center in before the practice, we should spend a few moments observing any physical or emotional changes. If we have created a new breath sequence, this time for observation gives us the opportunity to recognize whether the practice led us to our intended goal or if we need to make adjustments to the sequence. I generally practice a sequence four or five times, adjusting every time, until I feel like it does what I intended.

Once a breath sequence is created, it can be practiced as many times as is needed to fulfill your intention or bring you closer to your goal. Some sequences I do almost every day, like the Athletic Performance breath sequence (see pages 212 to 218). Others I do only when I feel a need. For example, if I am having difficulty sleeping, I do the Sleep sequence (see pages 199 to 205).

There is an old saying, "If you do nothing, nothing will happen." Unfortunately, this statement is untrue. If you do nothing, something *will* happen, but it probably won't be the outcome you want. Change is a universal truth. Everything is either growing or decaying. Growth is a result of activity; decay is a result of stagnation. Sometimes the path to positive change and growth isn't clear, and it might take some wandering to realize where you need to be. If you're unaware of where you are, where you came from, or the journey that led you here, how will you ever know what you need to do to manifest the change you desire?

Fortunately, with just a few conscious breaths of mindful awareness, you can observe the flow of your reality and recognize whether you are moving in the direction you want, fighting against an impossible current, or wasting away from stagnation. Science and philosophy can tell us only what we *should* be feeling or what *should* be happening; we still need to observe whether our intention comes to fruition. If we didn't get the results we were looking for, we know we need to course-correct.

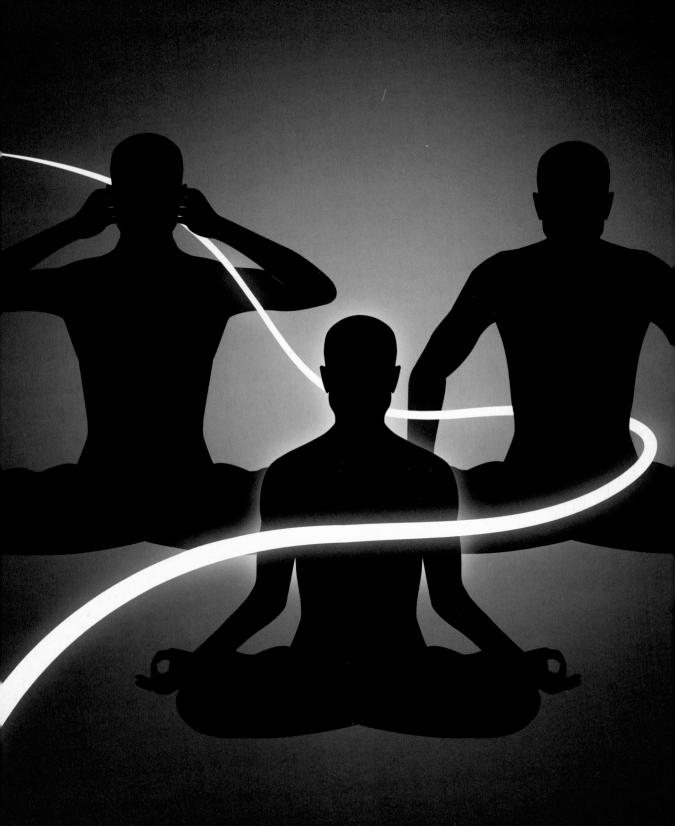

[SECTION 5]
BREATH-SEQUENCED THEMED PRACTICES

In this section, I've provided ten breath sequences that you can use, as well as explanations of how and why I structured the practices as I did. I hope these sequences give you more insight into how to use the breath as a powerful tool for physical, emotional, and spiritual change. You can use them to accomplish the stated goals or as examples to create your own breath sequences that serve your individual needs and manifest your personal goals.

The following sequences are at an intermediate difficulty. You may feel the need to lengthen or shorten some breath retentions or repetitions in order to make a practice more accessible or more challenging based on your personal goals.

Remember, the breath is a healing medicine. Each of these sequences serves as a different medication to use as needed, and as often as needed. Just like being prescribed a drug for an illness, taking one pill won't cure the ailment; we need to continue taking the medication until the problem is resolved or we receive the desired effect.

EQUANIMITY

This breath sequence focuses on creating a sense of balance and harmony between the mind, body, inner nature, and outer nature. It uses energy-balancing breathing practices that gradually increase in intensity while maintaining autonomic nervous system regularity. It then moves into balancing the emotions with the physical body, sustaining harmony with mild breath-holds, and ends with a slow energetic return to place the mind and body in a perfect state of serenity.

The state of equanimity centers on emotional and mental stability. While the quality is calm, it is the calmness that exists under tension and stress that makes this emotional and energetic state so vital. Equanimity is the keel on the hull of the sailboat that keeps the boat right even in the strongest winds and the most turbulent waves. It's the serenity we find in the eye of the storm; even if the world is falling apart, we remain unaffected. Our ability to maintain balance and harmony through the chaos and unforeseen challenges that life presents is the key to success and sanity. This breath sequence is meant to bring us back to our center if we are feeling either down and lethargic or stressed out and agitated.

To balance our autonomic nervous system, we want to stimulate the ventral vagal complex with our breathing. The ventral vagal complex is associated with the ability to interact with others in a healthy way and to handle tough situations without becoming overwhelmed or stressed out.

The *sattva guna* represents the equanimous state of balance and harmony and is energetically neutral. *Sattva* serves as the mode "to be," as in fully present and immersed in the now. To find emotional and energetic equanimity requires us to be in the present moment.

We also see an energetic balance with the *sushumna nadi* and the *prana vayu.* The *sushumna nadi* rises energetically from creating a balance between our passive, receptive side and our active, outgoing side. *Prana vayu* also focuses on the giving and receiving of energy and represents our inherent interconnectedness.

The equanimous mind and spirit come from the understanding that we are part of something bigger. We will always struggle to feel balanced when we think we are separate. Any form of separation presents itself as though something is missing; only by returning to the feeling of being whole can we know harmony.

As we move through the entirety of this sequence, we want to allow the breath to keep us centered, focused, and fully present. With the breath influencing balance through our energetic body, the intention to be here will manifest the goal of equanimity.

EQUANIMITY BREATH SEQUENCE
25 MINUTES

1:1 | INHALATION:EXHALATION	1:1:1:1 | INHALATION:INNER RETENTION:EXHALATION:OUTER RETENTION		
WARM-UP	***SAMA VRITTI*** **5:5 ➡ 15:15** Add 1 second per inhalation and exhalation per round up to 15:15 (5:5, 6:6, 7:7,...15:15)	1 ROUND	4–5 MINUTES (approximately)
HEAT-BUILDING	***NADI SHODHANA*** **WITH BOX BREATHING** **5:5:5:5**	20 ROUNDS	10 MINUTES (approximately)
VITALIZING	***VILOMA 3*** INHALATION: HOLD 3:2,2:3,1:4 EXHALATION: HOLD 1:4,2:3,3:2	20 ROUNDS	5 MINUTES (approximately)
COOL-DOWN	***SAMA VRITTI*** **15:15 ➡ 5:5** Subtract 1 second per inhalation and exhalation per round down to 5:5 (15:15, 14:14, 13:13,...5:5)	1 ROUND	5 MINUTES (approximately)

WARM-UP

The warm-up begins with *sama vritti pranayama* (see pages 114 to 117), creating a sense of balance through equal inhalations and exhalations. You maintain equal respirations but increase the duration of each respiration to increase the intensity of the practice gradually. The equality of the breath promotes *sattva guna* and regulates the autonomic nervous system. Lengthening each respiration enables you to slow your breathing and build up carbon dioxide, which stimulates the parasympathetic nervous system and promotes the feeling of calmness and relaxation. Slowly increasing the duration with each breath to the point that you experience a challenge ramps up the intensity and creates a sense of increased energy and readiness.

Start with a five-second inhalation followed by a five-second exhalation. With each progressing respiration, add one second to both parts of the breath. The second respiration is a six-second inhalation and a six-second exhalation. Continue until you reach fifteen seconds for the inhalation and exhalation for a total of eleven respirations (5:5, 6:6, 7:7,...15:15). When you inhale at the beginning of this warm-up, breathe only as deeply as you need for the duration of the breath. A five-second inhalation should be just slightly deeper than a normal inhalation, or approximately one-third of your vital capacity (full breath). As you progress through the warm-up, you will fill the lungs and expand the chest and belly a little more with each breath, slowly warming up the diaphragm and stretching the intercostal muscles.

HEAT-BUILDING

The heat-building component combines two breathing practices, *nadi shodhana* (see pages 132 to 136) and box breathing (see pages 114 to 117). These practices promote balance and harmony in slightly different ways. *Nadi shodhana* is an energetic harmonizing practice that focuses on creating unity through our polarizing qualities to restore balance. This exercise also balances the hemispheres of the mind. Box breathing increases heart rate variability and regulates the autonomic nervous system, stimulating the ventral vagal complex. Joining these practices accentuates their intention for creating balance, and because *nadi shodhana* leans more toward the energetic body and box breathing has a substantial impact on our physiological properties, combining the two techniques supports the intention of the mind-body connection.

Begin by placing your left hand in *jnana mudra* (wisdom *mudra*) on your left knee and taking *Vishnu mudra* (balancing *mudra*) with your right hand (see page 134). Close the right nostril with your right thumb, inhale for five seconds through the left nostril, and hold inner retention for five seconds, then close off the left nostril with your ring finger, exhale out the left nostril for five seconds, and hold outer retention for five seconds. Repeat this cycle, starting the second round with the inhalation through the right nostril. Continue for twenty rounds, or approximately ten minutes.

With this breath practice, the energy should remain relatively even. There is a slight build in intensity during the warm-up, with the longest respiration lasting about thirty seconds. Only the last five respirations of the warm-up are over twenty seconds. The heat-building practice is approximately a twenty-second-cycle breath, or three breaths per minute sustained for twenty minutes. Just like at the beginning of the warm-up, the inhalation is five seconds, so the breath should be slightly deeper than a regular inhalation, or approximately one-third of our vital capacity.

The box breathing component uses inner and outer retention. The retention is short, so it doesn't create too much of a challenge. Still, it does prepare us for the slightly more challenging retention that is in the vitalizing practice.

VITALIZING

The vitalizing component uses the *viloma* 3 *pranayama* unmodified (see pages 141 and 142). *Viloma* 3 balances the lengths and retention of the inhalation and exhalation, which creates a feeling of balance and equanimity, making it a great practice for our intention. It also stimulates the ventral vagal complex, increases heart rate variability, and promotes a *sattvic* state. If you follow the *viloma* 3 ratios of inhalation-to-retention 3:2, 2:3, 1:4 and exhalation-to-retention 1:4, 2:3, 3:2, each breath cycle is approximately thirty seconds, or two respirations per minute.

For many people, sustaining this practice for ten minutes is very challenging. You don't want this breath sequence practice to be too difficult, or it will increase *rajas* energy and pull you away from the intention. You should be able to maintain the practice for the duration of the sequence without feeling like you need to catch your breath (that breath hunger feeling). It's important to speed up the count so that the practice feels stimulating but not challenging so that you can maintain the sattvic energy.

COOL-DOWN

The cool-down is a mirror of the warm-up. Again, it uses *sama vritti* to maintain the balance of the autonomic nervous system and sustain the feeling of equanimity that was cultivated throughout the rest of the breath sequence. The cool-down starts with an inhalation-to-exhalation ratio of 15:15, or a thirty-second respiration. Because you are coming from the *viloma* 3 with a thirty-second respiration, the cool-down shouldn't feel like it is increasing in intensity. Each respiration shortens by one second per breath cycle. Slowly ramp down the duration and depth of the respirations until you reach a ratio of 5:5. Because each cycle is a little easier than the last, the intensity gradually decreases until you return to an effortless breath.

After the last breath of the sequence, remain with the intention and a normal, relaxed breath for a few moments. Notice the results of the practice and see if there are any changes or shifts in energy, mood, or feelings.

DEEP RELAXATION

This sequence focuses on slow breathing, gentle breath-holds, and practices that move toward feelings of relaxation and restoration to calm the mind, ease the nervous system, and fully let go to enjoy the present moment.

To experience a state of deep relaxation, we need to feel safe, both physically in our environment and emotionally in our sense of well-being. Any sense of fear or danger will inhibit our ability to relax. We don't need to be in danger to feel fear. And we obviously wouldn't do a deep relaxation breath sequence if there was an imminent threat. Fear arises from the unknown, from perceived danger that may or may not be real, but either way, our reaction is the same. Our fear might not present itself so obviously as us being scared of something, but more as a feeling of worry or stress—worry that we won't have enough money to pay the bills; concerns about our health, job, relationship, or family; apprehension about future endeavors; or a multiplicity of things. Often, these uncertainties repeat in the back of our minds, fueling the feelings of stress and anxiety, yet we ignore them as if they're normal. While it might be common, we are not meant to live under continuous stress.

When our minds are occupied with future events, future needs, and future self, we are prevented from experiencing the enjoyment of being fully present. Modern life encourages the hustle, and for most of us, it's a necessary part of life. Even if we are not stressed about being overloaded in our daily routine and we thrive on always being on the go, doing something or being a part of something, without rest we will eventually burn out. We can also try to be so busy that we feel like we have control of something because, in actuality, we feel like we are not in control. Releasing control might highlight the feeling of being out of control. Relaxation is necessary for the mind and body to repair themselves. However, most of us relax our bodies without ever resting our minds, so much so that our future projections creep into our dreams.

Fear, stress, worry, and the perpetual running of thoughts about what we need to do, accomplish, have, or become all arise from a perception of a future that may or may not happen. And while it is necessary to prepare for the future, we can only relax when we are present.

A common misconception is that we need to ignore the things that want to occupy our minds and consume our thoughts. The more we try to push them away, the more they will stand their ground. Instead, before this breath practice, take a moment to recognize and acknowledge your stream of thoughts, concerns, or needs. Only by bringing light to the situation can you see what is there. As thoughts enter the mind, let them come without resistance, without needing to change them or engage with them, and let them go when they no longer want to occupy your mind. As you move through the sequence, allow the breath to be your mantra. Let the breath come, let it be, and let it go. With it, the thoughts will follow, and you will experience a sense of being fully present.

DEEP RELAXATION BREATH SEQUENCE
27–30 MINUTES

	1:1 | INHALATION:EXHALATION	1:1:1 | INHALATION:INNER RETENTION:EXHALATION	
WARM-UP	**DIRGHA SVASAM 5:5** INHALATION: ABDOMEN 2 SECONDS, MID-CHEST 2 SECONDS, UPPER CHEST 1 SECOND EXHALATION: 5 SECONDS	30 ROUNDS (approximately)	5 MINUTES
HEAT-BUILDING	**RAMPED EXHALATION** 5:5 ➡ 5:15 INCREASE THE EXHALATION BY 1 SECOND PER ROUND UP TO A 15-SECOND EXHALATION (5:5, 5:6, 5:7,...5:15)	1 ROUND	2 MINUTES (approximately)
VITALIZING	**EXTENDED BREATH RETENTION** 5 SLOW BREATHS 30-SECOND INNER RETENTION 5 SLOW BREATHS 10-SECOND OUTER RETENTION	5–8 ROUNDS (approximately)	15 MINUTES
COOL-DOWN	**RELEASING BREATH** 10:10:SIGH 10:20:SIGH 10:30:SIGH Finish with relaxed natural breathing	1 ROUND	5 MINUTES

WARM-UP

The warm-up begins with *dirgha svasam pranayama* (see pages 104 to 107). The primary purpose of the three-part breathing exercise is to create a conscious connection between the mind, body, and breath while allowing the breath to keep you present. Here, slight modifications to *dirgha svasam* are made, adjusting the depth and effort of the breath to have a milder approach for the inhalation and fill only to 60 to 70 percent of your vital capacity. The inhalation is five seconds, with a ratio of 2:2:1. Inhale to expand the belly for two seconds, continue the inhalation to expand the mid-chest for two seconds, followed by the upper chest for one second, and conclude with an equal exhalation of five seconds. Equal respirations restore balance to the autonomic nervous system and promote the *sattvic* quality, "to be." You need to feel present to feel safe and let go of future thoughts and projections. The slower respiration rate of five to six breaths per minute produces a natural calming effect on the mind.

This breath practice can be done while seated or lying down. Sometimes lying down can be helpful in allowing the body to fully release control and relax, especially if you have a hard time surrendering. Placing one hand on the belly and one hand on the chest provides a touch that helps us feel connected and safe. Connecting your hands to your body also stimulates the peripheral nervous system to release tension in your muscles similar to the response your nervous system has while stretching your body.

Continue *dirgha svasam* for approximately five minutes. If you are still feeling anxious or if your mind is overactive, you can continue with this breath practice until you feel ready to move forward. Sometimes slow, relaxed, focused breathing is the best thing to release the mind from its busy nature.

HEAT-BUILDING

The heat-building component focuses on creating *tamasic* energy to build a sense of grounding and stability. The intensity of this breath increases slightly with every respiration cycle. As the intensity increases, the parasympathetic nervous system is stimulated, so you feel more relaxed even though the breath becomes more challenging. The warm-up flows directly into the heat-building component as you continue with the 5:5 ratio breathing but switches from the three-part breath to a natural inhalation where the chest and abdomen move in unison. With each respiration, add one second to the exhalation until you reach fifteen seconds (5:5, 5:6,

5:7,...5:15). This breath practice brings the focus to the exhalation. A longer exhalation-to-inhalation ratio contributes to feeling relaxed and at peace. Placing the focus on the exhalation moves with the letting go and grounding energy of *apana vayu*.

The heat-building component is relatively short, serving as a transition to the more challenging retention practice in the vitalizing component by lengthening the exhalation and slowly building up carbon dioxide.

VITALIZING

The vitalizing component brings the focus to creating an extended breath retention practice with relatively low difficulty. The intention is to sustain a retention practice, working through *antara kumbhaka* and *bahya kumbhaka*. You want to stimulate the dorsal vagal complex of the autonomic nervous system that fosters a sense of deep relaxation without triggering the sympathetic fight-or-flight response that could come from struggling to hold your breath.

After the final respiration of the heat-building component, transition to the vitalizing practice with five slow breaths. After the fifth breath, inhale deeply and hold inner retention for thirty seconds. After thirty seconds, exhale naturally and continue with five more slow breaths. After the fifth breath, exhale completely and hold the breath for a fifteen-second outer retention. The vitalizing practice continues by alternating between thirty-second inner retention and fifteen-second outer retention, with each hold separated by five slow breaths that enable recovery from the periods of retention. Try to breathe only as deeply as is needed, but if you are feeling challenged by the retention, take deeper breaths to help regulate your carbon dioxide levels or add a few more breaths to recover before continuing with the next retention.

This practice allows us to gradually increase our tolerance to carbon dioxide while slowly buffering our blood pH levels with intermittent breathing. Throughout the vitalizing component, the five slow, intermittent breaths become shallower and more effortless. The rise in carbon dioxide levels slows the heart, lowers blood pressure, opens the airway, and makes it easier to breathe while creating a state of deep relaxation.

Continue the breath cycle for fifteen to twenty minutes, or longer if you want or need to stay with it. If either the inner or outer retention feels too challenging, add more breaths between the holds. If it is still too difficult, shorten the length of the retention until it feels manageable.

COOL-DOWN

The cool-down focuses on complete surrender. The full cool-down is only three breaths followed by a short period of relaxed, natural breathing. Each of the three breaths has a ten-second inhalation followed by a progressively lengthening inner retention. The first retention is ten seconds, the second retention is twenty seconds, and the final retention is thirty seconds. After the hold, open your mouth and sigh deeply with a vocalized "ha." Sighing promotes a neurological response that releases stress and anxiety. This breathing exercise is about letting go and releasing control—releasing fears, stress, anxiety, and anything else you might be holding on to but is not providing you any benefit. With three deep breaths, let it all go.

After the third breath, let go of all control and return to normal, relaxed breathing. Release any thoughts, but don't try to push anything out. Whatever arises in your mind, let it come, let it be, and let it go. After a few minutes of resting in your natural breath, notice if anything is coming up as a result of the practice and see if there are any changes or shifts in energy, mood, or feelings.

ENERGY BOOST

This breath sequence focuses on practices that increase energy by stimulating the sympathetic nervous system and affecting the *rajas guna* as well as methods that facilitate cellular respiration and the production of ATP (energy). The sequence uses a combination of faster breathing exercises and moderate breath-holds as well as exercises that balance energy and increase our affect to connect socially.

There are many reasons we would want to do a practice to increase our energy levels, but probably the number one reason is that we feel a lack of energy or motivation and therefore need something to help us get moving. We naturally gravitate to laziness and lethargy, even though we know that chronic inactivity is one of the worst things for us. So why are we naturally lazy if it is so harmful? Modern life is about comfort. We live in a world where we can work, sleep, eat, shop, and enjoy countless hours of entertainment without ever leaving the couch. Things like food, water, warmth, safety, and shelter are standard commodities for the majority of people, but this wasn't always the case. People used to have to work for all these things. To procure water or make a fire took energy, to hunt and gather food took energy—every aspect of living required people to expel energy. If they used energy when it wasn't necessary to survive, they might not have had enough energy to catch their next meal. Resting and being inactive when moving wasn't required was essential for life. But now that activity is rarely needed, inactivity has become the default.

To move the body, sometimes we first need to energize the mind and awaken the spirit. When I was in the military, the word *motivation* was used often. We would go on motivational runs, yell motivational sayings, and sing motivational cadences to inspire ourselves to be eager to charge through the most difficult life-threatening situations or do uninspiring menial tasks without complaint. In that context, motivation meant brainwashing someone into wanting to do something they probably wouldn't otherwise want to do, like being willing to give your life for your country to support a cause you may not agree with. I have a different relationship to that word now. Today, I see motivation as the drive, the spark, the inspiration to carry out and fulfill my purpose and goals in life. But sometimes I recognize the need to want to do things I don't want to do. If my attitude is not in the place I need it to be, I have the breath to motivate me, to boost my energy and pull me out of whatever place I might feel stuck.

This breath practice awakens our inner fire to be the catalyst that sparks our motivation by stimulating the mobilization mechanisms of the autonomic nervous system so that we feel like we have the physical energy to get up and go. It does so by creating more sympathetic tone through intermittent rapid breathing exercises linked with breath retention to restore low carbon dioxide levels and increase cellular respiration, which produces more ATP (cellular energy). Throughout this sequence, we also work to improve our *rajas* energy by focusing on practices that are inhalation oriented.

Anytime the intention is to increase energy levels, we need to make sure that we maintain balance and establish practices that act as anchors or energy buffers. We want to stimulate the mind and body so we feel energized to work, play, and interact without creating feelings of restlessness or agitation. As we push the sympathetic nervous system, we must also maintain ventral vagal tone, the part of the sympathetic nervous system that facilitates our ability to interact socially. Again, we accomplish this by doing a breath sequence that works through balanced slow respirations, fast breathing exercises, and moderate breath retention.

ENERGY BOOST BREATH SEQUENCE
20 MINUTES

	1:1 | INHALATION:INNER RETENTION	1:1:1 | INHALATION:INNER RETENTION:EXHALATION	
WARM-UP	*UJJAYI PRANAYAMA* **10:5:5**	10 ROUNDS	3.5 MINUTES (approximately)
HEAT-BUILDING 1	**SLOW *BHASTRIKA* 30 SECONDS** INNER RETENTION 30 SECONDS **SLOW *BHASTRIKA* 30 SECONDS** INNER RETENTION 1 MINUTE	4 ROUNDS 1 ROUND	5 MINUTES (approximately)
HEAT-BUILDING 2	**FAST *BHASTRIKA* 15 SECONDS** OUTER RETENTION 15 SECONDS **FAST *BHASTRIKA* 15 SECONDS** OUTER RETENTION 30 SECONDS	5 ROUNDS 3 ROUNDS	5 MINUTES (approximately)
VITALIZING	*VILOMA 1* INHALATION: HOLD 3:2, 2:3, 1:4 EXHALATION: 5 SECONDS	15 ROUNDS	5 MINUTES (approximately)
COOL-DOWN	*SITALI PRANAYAMA* INHALATION: 10 SECONDS INNER RETENTION: 15 SECONDS LION'S BREATH EXHALATION	5 ROUNDS	1.5 MINUTES (approximately)

WARM-UP

The warm-up utilizes a strong *ujjayi* breath (see pages 108 to 113) to build internal heat and stimulate your inner *agni* (fire) energy. *Rajas* energy, which is the *guna* associated with passion, drive, and obtaining goals, is stimulated by increasing the inhalation to twice the exhalation length. To prevent overstimulation of the sympathetic nervous system while still in the warm-up, inner retention is added to match the exhalation. The inner retention slows the breath and accentuates the length of the inhalation both to give you more of the energetic feeling that you experience from an inhalation-focused breath practice and to maintain balanced carbon dioxide levels.

    The respirations for this practice consist of a ten-second inhalation, a five-second inner retention, and a five-second exhalation. You can increase the intensity of the warm-up by lengthening each component, keeping the ratio of 2:1:1, and still get the same intended effect from the practice. With the ten-second inhalation (or longer if you choose a longer breath ratio), work to fully expand the lungs to strengthen the diaphragm and stretch the intercostal muscles. The exhalations are forceful with a strong contraction of the core. Keep the exhalation slow by increasing the constriction of the throat; this also makes the sound of the breath more pronounced. Continue the breath cycle for ten respirations.

HEAT-BUILDING

The heat-building component consists of two similar exercises that progress in intensity. The first exercise starts with a slow *bhastrika* breath at a rate of one full respiration per second for thirty seconds. *Bhastrika* (see pages 126 to 128) uses the power of the core to pump the breath in and out, further stimulating inner fire and strengthening the stomach. During the thirty-second *bhastrika* breath, you are blowing off carbon dioxide and elevating your blood pH to stimulate the sympathetic nervous system. The rapid breathing is immediately followed by a thirty-second inner retention. During the retention, you might feel some of the invigorating effects of hyperventilating, such as light-headedness and tingling in the fingers, face, and belly. This is a common effect of hyperventilation and a good sign that you are blowing off lots of carbon dioxide. The thirty-second retention is not long enough for you to return to baseline, so you start the second round slightly hypocapnic. Repeat the first breath, with the *bhastrika* and the retention. When you get to the third breath, you are even more carbon dioxide deficient, which should make the final one-minute hold relatively easy.

After the third round of the first heat-building component, double the speed of the *bhastrika* breath to approximately two breaths per second. You want to keep the same depth and drive of the breath, utilizing the power of the core and diaphragm to move as much air per breath as possible. After fifteen seconds, or about thirty *bhastrika* breaths, hold outer retention for fifteen seconds. Continue this cycle of fifteen-second rapid abdominal breathing and fifteen-second outer retention for five rounds. As with the first *bhastrika* breath, with each cycle you become slightly more hypocapnic. After five rounds, continue with three more rounds with a thirty-second outer retention. Hopefully, at this stage, you have expelled enough carbon dioxide that the first thirty-second retention is relatively easy. The second and third rounds might be slightly harder. You want to experience mild breath hunger by the last retention. If you are not feeling it, you can hold the final retention for a minute to build your carbon dioxide levels back up. For most people, thirty seconds should be sufficient to prepare for the vitalizing component.

The breath retention helps balance excessive stimulation of the sympathetic nervous system and limits the other adverse physiological effects from rapid breathing. The outer retention works to decrease blood saturation and stimulate red blood cell production. Outer retention accomplishes this more quickly than inner retention because there is less oxygen in the lungs, and therefore it is easier to decrease oxygen levels. Increasing the percentage of red blood cells increases VO_2 max and your overall energy levels even after sympathetic tone comes down.

VITALIZING

The vitalizing component's primary purpose is to maintain and support the cultivated *rajas* energy from the previous exercises while stabilizing the autonomic nervous system and increasing cellular respiration for the production of more ATP (cellular energy) for the body to utilize. The *viloma* 1 *pranayama* practice (see pages 137 to 139) creates many of the desired effects that you need to accomplish the goal of this component. *Viloma* 1 inhalation and retention are each twice the exhalation, which promotes *rajas* energy. The interrupted inhalation stimulates the mind and breaks normal breathing patterns, increasing cognitive awareness. This practice follows the breath ratio of 3:2, 2:3, 1:4:5—three-second belly inhalation, two-second inner retention, two-second mid-chest inhalation, three-second inner retention, one-second upper chest inhalation, four-second inner retention, and five-second exhalation.

A strong *ujjayi* technique is incorporated into the interrupted inhalation and exhalation. Just like in the warm-up, using this powerful breath continues to stoke your inner fire, increasing internal heat and energy and raising your *rajas guna*. The *ujjayi* breath also helps regulate the duration of each part of the inhalation, adding an extra level of control and mindfulness. The *viloma* 1 retention practice may also effect a splenic contraction, increasing the amount of circulating red blood cells, which will deliver more oxygen for cellular respiration and energy production.

COOL-DOWN

The cool-down uses the cooling *sitali* breath to balance any excessive heat generated from the other practices in this sequence. *Sitali* is a technique that involves inhaling through the mouth with the tongue curled like a tube or straw (see pages 148 and 149). The air passes over the tongue, and cool air enters the lungs. While this practice uses this breath to cool the body, it is modified by lengthening the inhalation to ten seconds to maintain *rajas* energy. The inhalation is followed by a fifteen-second breath retention to slow the breath rate and allow you to continue the breath retention benefits as you come to the close of the practice. The exhalation uses a breath technique called *simhasana,* or lion's breath, which is briefly mentioned on page 149. Lion's breath is an open-mouth exhalation where you extend the tongue toward your chin and look up toward the third eye area while making an aspirated "ha" sound. It is a fantastic exercise that invigorates the muscles of the face and tongue.

While it might feel silly to suck air through your tongue like a straw and then stick out your tongue and say "ha" while rolling your eyes back in your head, this technique has several physiological benefits. The intention is to increase energy, but you want to do so in a way that doesn't spark a fight-or-flight response. You want to have the energy to move, work, interact, and play. Finding this balance requires the healthy activation of the dorsal vagal complex. One thing that we haven't discussed about the polyvagal theory is how the cranial nerves influence the ventral and dorsal vagal complexes and our ability to engage socially and feel safe. Of the twelve pairs of cranial nerves, the majority link to the movement of our facial muscles, tongue, and eyes. Exercising the movements between *sitali pranayama* and lion's breath stimulates many of the cranial nerves that influence the ventral and dorsal vagal complexes, increasing our energy while regulating the sympathetic nervous system.

Note: The polyvagal theory is a complex subject, so my intention is to give you a digestible and usable understanding of it in relation to breathing. If you're interested in learning more about this revolutionary theory, I suggest that you check out the work of Dr. Stephen Porges and Stanley Rosenberg.

STRESS AND ANXIETY RELIEF

This breath sequence focuses on creating a feeling of balance and harmony and alleviating stress and anxiety through practices that promote the *sattva* and *tamas gunas* by using mild breathing methods and gentle breath-holds. It also utilizes techniques that make the autonomic nervous system more resilient to stress-induced responses so that when we face situations that would typically create stress, we can remain calm and centered.

Life can be arduous. We are constantly challenged, tested, and pushed to our limits. Stress might come from work, financial difficulties, or contention with a friend, family member, or loved one. Sometimes the feeling is more than stress; it's something that arises from within us, causing anguish and suffering that we can't seem to shake. When we face stressful situations, we might take that stress upon ourselves, but generally, as the situation changes or dissipates, the feelings that accompany it also leave. But if the feeling is coming from inside, changing external circumstances will not liberate us from the darkness.

Stress is caused by external factors and, if left unchecked, can cause serious health problems, weaken the immune system, and lead to over-eating, under-eating, muscle pain, insomnia, depression, and anxiety. Stress also affects how we act, react, and treat people. When we're under high levels of stress, we can be very emotional, irritable, angry, fearful, and insecure and react in ways that are not normal for us. If chronic stress is not rectified, then even when the external stress-causing factors are removed, the internal affliction can remain.

Anxiety is slightly different. Although it is often a result of stress, it comes from within. Anxiety can be caused by genetics, altered brain chemistry, or severe life-changing events. It can create all the physical and mental health problems that we get from stress and develop into more severe conditions such as panic attacks, post-traumatic stress disorder (PTSD), phobias, and social anxiety. If you already suffer from an anxiety disorder, then you are well aware of the foreboding feelings that accompany it.

Breath practices can immediately improve how we feel and diminish stress and anxiety. While breathing exercises might not provide an immediate cure to chronic anxiety disorders, they can definitely help, especially when accompanied by meditation and therapy.

Stress should subside when we leave behind the situation that is causing stress. However, we can physically leave but mentally and emotionally carry the stress with us. We see this when we bring our work problems home and allow work stress to affect our personal life. If our stress is generated from something like financial problems, relationship problems, or an event from the past, then we might not be able to leave or change our situation. Still, we can choose how we see the situation, how we let the situation affect us, and how we view ourselves as a part of that situation.

After I returned from fighting in the Iraq War at the end of 2003, I developed PTSD. I had nightmares and difficulty sleeping. I felt super anxious and always on guard. I would have occasional panic attacks, which I hadn't experienced since I was a child. The worst part was that I felt numb and disconnected from my friends and family. My more severe symptoms faded with time, and whatever was left, I pushed down and buried deep inside me. Unfortunately, I didn't get rid of it; I just hid it. I ended up carrying my past trauma with me much longer than I realized, and it continued to affect me long after I thought it was gone.

When I developed a meditation and yoga practice, I was able to recognize the deep pain that I had been carrying, not just from my experience in the war but from my childhood and everything else. My practice helped me to see the truth: that I was not my past, and my present life was beautiful. I was able to find gratitude for my past, how it led me here, and how those situations formed who I am. I had a new story, and I was a different person. My past life could not control who my future self would be.

If we make dough and bake it into bread, the bread will never be dough again; it is something completely different. Bread doesn't go around thinking that it's dough just because it used to be dough, and we don't need to live in the past just because we came from our past. Our breath is a constant reminder to be present and a powerful tool to let go of anything that is causing stress or anxiety.

Note: The breath is fantastic for releasing feelings of stress and anxiety, but if your symptoms are chronic and debilitating, then I encourage you to seek professional help. Anxiety-related disorders are highly treatable, yet few people who suffer from them seek professional help.

STRESS AND ANXIETY RELIEF BREATH SEQUENCE
10–12 MINUTES

	1:1 | INHALATION:EXHALATION 1:1:1 | INHALATION: INNER RETENTION:EXHALATION		
WARM-UP	***SAMA VRITTI* (PYRAMID RATIO)** **0 ➡ 1:1 1:1 ➡ 10:1** Increase each respiration by 1 up to 10:10 Decrease each respiration by 1 down to 1:1 (1:1, 2:2,...10:10, 9:9, 8:8,...1:1)	1 ROUND	4 MINUTES (approximately)
HEAT-BUILDING	**BREATH OF FIRE** (15 RESPIRATIONS) INNER RETENTION: 5 SECONDS EXHALATION: OPEN-MOUTH SIGH	5 ROUNDS	2 MINUTES (approximately)
VITALIZING	**4:7:8 BREATH** Inhalation: 4 seconds Inner retention: 7 seconds Pursed-lip exhalation: 8 seconds	5 ROUNDS	2 MINUTES (approximately)
COOL-DOWN	**TWO-PART-RATIO BREATH** **10:10:2|2:10:10** 10-second inhalation, 10-second inner retention, 2-second exhalation, 2-second inhalation, 10-second inner retention, and 10-second exhalation	5 ROUNDS	4 MINUTES (approximately)

WARM-UP

The warm-up begins by settling into a natural breath. Think of something you are grateful for and hold that gratitude in your heart as you breathe. Gratitude is one of the most powerful practices for overcoming stress and anxiety. Our intention for the warm-up is to bring awareness to the breath through an exercise that is less challenging and requires some focus and awareness to keep us present. The breath needs to be calming and promote balanced *sattva* energy while giving us a sense of control and stability. We want to slowly ramp up the intensity and warm up the lungs and respiratory muscles with gradually deepening breaths.

This component uses *sama vritti* (see pages 114 to 117), adding a pyramid-style ratio to build the breath practice. Begin with a very light, soft breath of 1:1, barely filling the lungs or using any effort. With each complete respiration, add one second until you reach 10:10. With each breath, you also want to breathe slightly deeper. Once you reach the ten-second inhalation and ten-second exhalation, subtract one second, working back down to 1:1 and decreasing in depth and intensity. Starting from a simple, effortless breath and building up to something more challenging but still manageable and then returning to a calm, effortless breath begins to train the mind to feel challenged without being stressed. If you are coming into this practice feeling anxious, you might feel that anxiety throughout the warm-up, and that's okay. You can repeat the warm-up if you feel like it will help or move on to the heat-building section.

HEAT-BUILDING

The heat-building component uses breath of fire (see pages 129 to 131) to stimulate the sympathetic nervous system without provoking the fight-or-flight response that we often feel when we are stressed. Breath of fire is a rapid, smooth, shallow, almost effortless practice, which is different from the type of hyperventilation that often accompanies an anxiety attack, where the breath is rapid, deep, effortful, and uncontrollable. In this practice, breath of fire is fifteen quick respirations lasting seven to ten seconds, followed by a deep inhalation with a five-second hold and an open-mouth exhalation. Repeat this cycle five times. Keeping the rounds of breath of fire short and following them with breath retention limits the effects of hypocapnia that might be invoked by a sustained breath of fire practice or a *pranayama* technique such as *kapalabhati* or *bhastrika,* which requires more effort and expels more carbon dioxide.

The rapid breathing stimulates our *rajas guna,* giving us an energetic boost and loosening areas of tension. Since any fast breathing can feel similar to what we experience when we feel panic, this technique quickly interrupts the rapid breath with a deep inhalation and brief hold to establish a sense of control and give a feeling of relief. The breath-hold is followed by an open-mouth exhalation that allows us to release all the built-up stress and anxiety that we might be carrying. This technique strengthens the autonomic nervous system to be more resilient against a stress-induced response. By establishing control and alleviating built-up tension, we can transition the sympathetic nervous system from an unsafe response that triggers fight-or-flight to a safe response that supports interaction and connection.

VITALIZING

The vitalizing component uses 4-7-8 breath (see page 120), which therapists commonly employ to help patients relax. The practice is based on *vishama vritti,* an unequal ratio breathing practice (see pages 118 to 121), with a modification to the exhalation. The ratio of inhalation to exhalation is 1:2, which cultivates *tamasic* energy and stimulates the parasympathetic nervous system. The breath retention and slow respiratory rate of three breaths per minute slowly build up carbon dioxide levels, which slows the heart rate, lowers blood pressure, and relaxes the mind and body. What makes this practice unique is the pursed-lip exhalation. Pursed-lip breathing is something that emphysema patients do to increase the pressure inside their lungs and keep the alveolar sacs from collapsing due to the lack of surfactant caused by the disease. By doing the same thing, we can expand into the deeper areas of the lungs and push more oxygen into the cells. Pursed-lip breathing also stimulates the vagus nerve. Studies have shown that pursed-lip breathing encourages relaxation and, through stimulation of the autonomic nervous system, improves cardiorespiratory physiological functions.[1]

The 4-7-8 breath is easy to do and can be done as a stand-alone practice anytime you feel stressed and need to relax. Start with a four-second inhalation through the nose, and then hold the breath for seven seconds, followed by an eight-second pursed-lip exhalation. When you exhale, make your mouth small like you are whistling or holding a straw in your lips. The exhalation should be strong enough that you feel the increased pressure in your chest but not so strong that it feels forced, like blowing on hot soup, not like blowing out birthday candles. Repeat this exercise for five cycles.

COOL-DOWN

The cool-down is a two-part-ratio breath practice that alternates between emphasizing the inhalation and the exhalation. This practice intends to create a balanced, harmonious *sattvic* state by varying the stimulation of the sympathetic nervous system and the parasympathetic nervous system. Stress and anxiety can push us toward feelings of agitation and restlessness or feelings of depression and weakness. It doesn't matter whether we activate the sympathetic nervous system or the parasympathetic nervous system if it is coming from a place of unease. Both sides are creating a negative stress response, either fight-or-flight or freeze. Here, we use the breath to establish a sense of safety and care. Then, by strengthening both sides of the autonomic nervous system separately while creating balance, we can move out of both negative states into a place of tranquility.

The breath practice alternates between breath rates of 10:10:2 and 2:10:10. The first part of the sequence brings the focus to the inhalation and is more sympathetic. The second part brings attention to the exhalation and is more parasympathetic. We start with a ten-second inhalation, a ten-second inner retention, and a two-second full exhalation, followed by a two-second full inhalation, a ten-second inner retention, and a ten-second exhalation. After the first breath, the transition between the first exhalation and the second inhalation feels very quick. However, when we get to the third breath, we are following a long exhalation with another long inhalation. The long breaths give us a feeling of relaxation, and the short breaths give us a feeling of relief and ease, dissolving any pressure or worry.

SLEEP

This breath sequence works to clear the mind, calm the nervous system, and promote a state of deep relaxation for sound, healthy sleep. It uses breath practices that create a meditation object to liberate the mind from busy or worrisome thoughts that keep us awake. It also uses techniques that balance the hemispheres of the brain, energetically neutralizing the mind while stimulating neurotransmitters that promote deep quality sleep. This short, effortless sequence enables us to wind down, let go, and prepare for a restful, rejuvenating night.

There are five factors we can control that have the greatest impact on our health:

- How much we sleep

- How we breathe

- What we eat and drink

- How much we exercise

- How we handle stress

Most people give merit to only two, diet and exercise, and I definitely used to be a part of that group.

At the age of eighteen, I started down a path of sleep deprivation. When I was in the Marine Corps (a branch of the United States military), we trained to be able to handle sleep deprivation. During my six months in Iraq, I don't think I ever slept more than four hours a night. After I left the Marines, I worked for several years on ambulances and in an emergency room. I always worked the night shift because it paid more, and at that time, money was more important to me than sleep. On the nights that I worked, I would either take a short nap before my shift or just stay up all day and night, because I also wanted a social life. Sometimes I would follow my 7 p.m.-to-7 a.m. shift with another twelve-hour day shift to maximize the overtime pay, and the hospital didn't seem to mind if their healthcare staff worked twenty-four hours straight without breaks or sleep—in fact, they encouraged it because they were often so short-staffed. Many night shift workers are sleep-deprived zombies, hyped up on caffeine, and I lived on energy drinks.

When I became a firefighter, my normal shift was two days on, four days off. During the two working days, we slept at night unless there were emergencies that we needed to respond to. I often went forty-eight to seventy-two hours (if I picked up an overtime shift) with little to no sleep because we would be up all night running calls. There is a reason why many firefighters die in their fifties and sixties. Sleeping less than six hours a night regularly is a huge detriment to your health and makes you 200 percent more likely to die of a heart attack or stroke.[2]

Although I was physically fit and ate a proper diet (minus the copious amounts of caffeine), I frequently got sick and always had cold sores, which are a sign of a weak immune system. I was young, so I felt like I could handle a consistent lack of sleep. I subscribed to the "I'll sleep when I'm dead" motto. Unfortunately, sleep is neither optional nor negotiable. Sleep is a necessary and crucial biological function that supports our immune system, brain functions and emotional stability, metabolism and insulin levels, and heart health. Without proper sleep, we are more likely to get sick and develop heart disease and diabetes, and our risk of cancer increases significantly. Lack of sleep also reduces our ability to think and learn. We become more prone to accidents, and our sex drive suffers. The list of adverse effects goes on. Most sleep experts agree that adults need seven to nine hours of sleep a night, and children need even more. On top of getting an adequate amount of sleep, we need good-quality sleep.

I make sleep a priority and try to get at least eight hours a night. I use a device to measure how fast I fall asleep, how much REM and deep sleep I get, my body temperature, and my heart rate variability. By tracking my sleep, I can see how things like diet, exercise, and stress affect the quality of my sleep and ultimately my health, because sleep and health are so closely related.

Here are some things you can do to improve your quality and duration of sleep:

- **Don't have caffeine after 11 a.m. and limit your daily caffeine consumption.** Caffeine keeps us awake because it blocks the chemical adenosine, which makes us feel sleepy. The more caffeine we consume, the longer it takes for the body to process. Caffeine has a half-life of about five to six hours.[3] A single cup of coffee has about 100 milligrams (mg) of caffeine. You will still have about 50 mg of caffeine in your system at noon from that 7 a.m. cup of joe. But if you drink three cups of coffee in the morning (300 mg), you'll still have 50mg of caffeine flowing through your veins at 8 p.m.

- **Do not eat for at least four hours before going to bed.** When I eat late, I wake up often throughout the night. Digestion requires a ton of energy and extra blood in our digestive organs. This elevates our heart rate and makes us more restless throughout the night.

- **Keep a consistent bedtime.** Since I am consistently traveling around the world, I often have to battle with jet lag, different time zones, and an altered sleep schedule. Dealing with jet lag is difficult, but I have developed a few healthy ways to cope with it, such as allowing myself a few days to naturally adjust to the time difference before I do something that would require me to wake up early and interrupt my sleep. I never take sleeping medications to try and speed up the adjustment period. They are not as helpful as some people think. Sleeping medicine is also incredibly unhealthy, highly addictive, and results in poor-quality sleep.

- **Limit your exposure to blue light after sundown and dim lighting a few hours before your bedtime.** The blue light emitted from screens and lights can trick your body into thinking it's daytime and make it difficult to fall asleep. There are apps for your computer and phone, as well as settings on your television, that change your screens to amber light. You can also wear blue-blocking glasses after the sun goes down. Overhead lighting also fools the body into thinking it's daytime. Turn off overhead lights and use dim table lights or candles.

- **Exercise in the morning or afternoon.** When I work out in the evening, it's harder for me to fall asleep. Working out increases sympathetic tone, heart rate, and body temperature, all things we want to subdue before trying to sleep. It's recommended not to engage in rigorous physical activity for at least two hours before bedtime.

- **Limit alcohol consumption.** I notice a massive difference in my sleep when I drink alcohol versus when I don't. The liver needs time to metabolize the alcohol in the body, which can lead to sleep disruptions. The quality of sleep also goes down considerably. While we may feel like it's easier to sleep because alcohol is a sedative, the same sedation also impairs REM and deep sleep, leaving us with a long night of poor-quality light sleep. If you are going to drink in the evening, try to limit the number of drinks and stop at least four hours before your bedtime to allow your body time to process the alcohol.

- **Don't use an alarm clock to wake up.** If you need an alarm clock to rouse you, you're not getting enough sleep. Make your bedtime earlier so that you can wake up naturally with a full night's sleep, even if a situation requires you to wake up abnormally early. It's difficult for most people with good sleep habits to oversleep.

- **Do *pranayama* in bed before going to sleep.** For some people, meditation can be beneficial at night. However, I find *pranayama* much more effective. I don't meditate before going to sleep. I like to meditate in the morning when I feel the most alert. I don't want to train my body to feel sleepy when I do a mediation practice, but this is my personal preference. *Pranayama,* however, is a great tool to prepare the mind and body for a good night's sleep.

Many of us struggle to fall asleep or stay asleep because we haven't let go of the day. We are still thinking about our stresses and worries or about what we need to do the following day. Even if we limit alcohol and caffeine and do all the other things listed above to help improve our sleep, we have to quiet our minds and calm our emotions to enjoy a restful night. The breath can clear the mind, bring us back to the present moment, and release stress. The practices in this breath sequence help suppress the sympathetic nervous system and decrease stress hormones while increasing parasympathetic tone to promote rest and deep sleep. As you move through the sequence, if at any time you feel like lying down and falling asleep, it's okay to stop.

After completing the breath sequence, you can continue doing the cool-down breath until you drift off, or you can release the practice entirely. If it takes you longer than twenty minutes to fall asleep, try getting up and doing something relaxing for a little bit. Lying in bed trying to sleep can feel like torture. You can also take a cool shower and then repeat this practice. Cool showers are my go-to when I am really struggling to fall asleep. Lowering your body temperature helps promote sleep. If it takes you longer than thirty minutes to fall asleep, it's a sign that you are not getting enough sleep, and you already have a sleep deficit. In the morning, look at the list presented earlier and see if there is anything that you can change to help you relax and reclaim your sleep.

SLEEP SEQUENCE 10 MINUTES			
1:1 | INHALATION:EXHALATION		1:1:1 | INHALATION:INNER RETENTION:EXHALATION	
WARM-UP	**SAMA VRITTI (3-PART RAMPED RATIO)** **5:5:5 ➡ 10:10:10** Increase each ratio breath by 1 second from 5:5:5 to 10:10:10 (5:5:5, 6:6:6, 7:7:7...10:10:10)	1 ROUND	2 MINUTES (approximately)
HEAT-BUILDING	**NADI SHODHANA 6:12 WITH** **BHRAMARI ON THE EXHALATION**	5 ROUNDS	3 MINUTES (approximately)
VITALIZING	**VISHAMA VRITTI 4:6:10**	15 ROUNDS	5 MINUTES (approximately)
COOL-DOWN	**NATURAL, EFFORTLESS BREATHING** (LYING DOWN)	AS NEEDED	AS NEEDED

WARM-UP

The warm-up begins in a comfortable seated position, preferably where you intend to sleep. Take a few moments to feel the natural rhythm of your breath. This breath practice uses a variation of *sama vritti,* an easier method of box breathing that skips the more challenging outer retention and promotes a state of deep relaxation by stimulating the parasympathetic nervous system and slowly increasing carbon dioxide levels. Start with a five-second inhalation, a five-second inner retention, and a five-second exhalation and gradually lengthen the duration of each part of the breath to ease into the practice. As in other similar practices, you only want to inhale to about a third of your vital capacity. With each breath cycle, add one second to the three-part equal breath ratio and deepen the inhalation until you reach a thirty-second breath cycle of 10:10:10 (i.e., 5:5:5, 6:6:6, 7:7:7,...10:10:10). When you reach the ten-second ratio, fill your lungs only about two-thirds of your full breath, or to the point right before it feels effortful to continue inhaling.

This rhythmic, repetitive, sequential breath counting gives the mind a task to free it from other thoughts that might be keeping you awake. Counting the breath during *pranayama* is similar to using the breath as a meditation object. The breath keeps you present so that your mind is not drawn to the thoughts and stories that occupy it. The practice should feel relaxed. If you find the last few cycles challenging, you can adjust the count to start lower and lengthen it to where you feel comfortable.

HEAT-BUILDING

The heat-building component combines a few breathing techniques to support the intention of balancing the mind, increasing nitric oxide levels to help induce sleep, promote relaxation, and cultivate calming *tamasic* energy. *Nadi shodhana pranayama* (see pages 132 to 136) acts like an energetic twist for the mind, creating a balance between the right and left hemispheres of the brain while neutralizing our thoughts. To create relaxing *tamasic* energy and stimulate the parasympathetic nervous system, use a 1:2 breath ratio. I suggest a six-second inhalation and a twelve-second exhalation. If that ratio feels challenging to you, however, try 5:10 or 4:8. Because you want it to remain fairly effortless, you don't need to extend the duration of the breath by too much. You also add *bhramari pranayama* (see pages 144 to 147) to the exhalation to increase nitric oxide levels. Nitric oxide improves sleep quality and duration and promotes REM and deep sleep, which are necessary for brain function and memory consolidation.

Start the breath practice with a six-second inhalation through the right nostril while closing off the left nostril. Then switch, closing off the right nostril and exhaling out the left nostril for twelve seconds while making the sound "om," or a nasal humming sound. Continue this breath with a six-second inhalation through the right nostril and a twelve-second *bhramari* exhalation out the left nostril. When you finish the exhalation on the left side, you have completed one cycle. After five cycles, move on to the vitalizing component.

VITALIZING

The vitalizing component uses a breath ratio with a long exhalation that is equal to the combined duration of the inhalation and inner retention to foster calming *tamasic* energy while promoting a sense of balanced *sattvic* energy. As you come into this part of the breath practice, I suggest lying on your back and resting your hands on your belly and chest or alongside your body. Inhale equally into your chest and abdomen for four seconds so that both expand at the same rate. Breathe as deeply as feels comfortable. Hold your breath for six seconds, followed by a slow, controlled ten-second exhalation. Repeat this breath for about five minutes. If you feel like you want to let go of the breath control at any time, feel free to release this practice and move on to the cool-down.

COOL-DOWN

The cool-down returns you to your natural, effortless breath. Release all control of your breathing and let your body take over. Feel the cadence that the breath creates, its natural rhythm. You can spend a few moments observing the sensations of the breath or release your mind completely. Scan your body, starting at the head. Systematically relax each body part. It helps to gently engage the muscles in the area of focus before fully releasing them. Start by relaxing your face and jaw, then relax your shoulders and upper and lower arms. Release your hands. Relax your chest and soften your belly. Relax your legs and feet. Do a quick body scan to see if you are still holding on to any tension. You can remain on your back or slowly move into a more comfortable sleeping position.

CONCENTRATION AND MEMORY

This breath sequence intends to create mental stability, balance the hemispheres of the brain, and boost our ability to concentrate while limiting our tendency to be distracted. Through several breathing techniques, we increase attentiveness, decrease stress hormones, and generate a massive boost of nitric oxide. One of the many benefits of nitric oxide is its effectiveness as a neurotransmitter, which functions to boost our mental clarity, thought fluency, creativity, and ability to retain knowledge.

The mind is like any other muscle; to function optimally, it must be exercised. We wouldn't do well if we tried to run a marathon without training for it. Similarly, if we don't train the mind, it becomes weak, lazy, impulsive, and easily distracted. If we want to be able to focus our thoughts, direct our attention, expand our creativity, and increase our capacity to learn and remember complex ideas and information, we need to understand the tool that we are using to accomplish these things. The mind is the most powerful and complex tool at our disposal, yet most of us aren't aware of how little control we have of our mind or how to regain that control. Distractions, emotions, and anxiety affect our ability to concentrate, learn, and form new memories.

I used to spend a lot of time creating distractions. I called it multitasking, but multitasking is just an exploitation of our inability to maintain focus on a singular task. I remember times when I would be sitting on the couch simultaneously watching television, texting on my phone, and scrolling the internet on my computer. When I needed to focus on something or be creative, my mind would seek out every distraction it could find, because I had trained it to be distracted.

If we try to read something but keep switching our attention to something else and then return to what we were reading, we will probably have to go back and reread what we have already read. Our inability to stay focused on one task is a massive waste of time. To concentrate on one thing, the brain uses its working memory. If we are constantly switching between tasks, the mind has to dump the previous task and reload the new one into its working memory. The more we do that, the less productive the mind is, and the more time it takes to accomplish each task. We might call it multitasking, but multitasking is a misnomer. We are rapidly switching singular tasks, and each switch comes with a penalty, both in the time it takes to refocus and in our ability to retain information.

Attention is a limited resource that the mind allocates to the things it thinks are the most important. If we don't assign to it what is essential, then the mind will continue to search for something that it thinks is more relevant to the situation. Attention comes from intention. Clear intention lets the mind know what we consider to be the most important. Our intention illuminates the path along which we want our attention to follow. The clearer the path, the easier it is for the mind to stay on task. When we understand the ways in which the mind wants to wander, we are quicker at redirecting it when it strays. Life is the direct result of where we focus our attention. If we cannot direct our attention to manifest our purpose and desires, then life becomes very challenging.

One of the most effective and powerful ways to train the mind is through meditation and *pranayama*. Meditation is the process of observing the mind and noticing how it moves, what it is attracted to, and how to bring it back to a seemingly uninteresting task, like being aware of the breath. Obviously, there is much more to meditation; however, to understand the mind, we need to step back and observe what it naturally does. We may never truly comprehend the mind, but that doesn't mean we shouldn't try. Trying to fully understand the mind is like searching for the end of the universe: we'll never find it, but our search deepens our understanding of it and so much more. Only through broadening our awareness can we hope to gain a better perspective on what we know or think is true. Our perspective leads to clarity, which creates creativity, and I feel that being able to harness the mind's creativity is one of the greatest gifts the mind has to offer.

The breath is more powerful than just giving the mind something to focus on during meditation. The breath has the ability to influence our energy so that we are more alert and it's easier to focus, as well as stabilizing our emotions and neutralizing feelings of stress and anxiety, making it easier to learn and form new memories. We can use the breath to balance the hemispheres of our brain, which enables creativity. Through breathing, we can increase the production and absorption of nitric oxide, a powerful neurotransmitter that increases mental clarity and the ability to learn and retain information. As stated earlier in this book, the mind follows the breath. If we want to harness the power of the mind, we need to wield the power of the breath.

CONCENTRATION AND MEMORY BREATH SEQUENCE
20–25 MINUTES

1:1:1 | INHALATION:EXHALATION:OUTER RETENTION		1:1:1:1 | INHALATION:INNER RETENTION:EXHALATION:OUTER RETENTION		
WARM-UP	**BOX BREATHING 5:5:5*:5** **BHRAMARI PRANAYAMA* ON EXHALATION	15 ROUNDS	5 MINUTES (approximately)	
HEAT-BUILDING	*BHASTRIKA* **30 SECONDS**	6 ROUNDS	5 MINUTES	
VITALIZING	*VISHAMA VRITTI* **10:20:10*:5** **BHRAMARI PRANAYAMA* ON EXHALATION	6–12 ROUNDS	5 TO 10 MINUTES	
COOL-DOWN	*NADI SHODHANA* **10:10*:5** INHALATION: 10 SECONDS **BHRAMARI* EXHALATION: 10 SECONDS OUTER RETENTION: 5 SECONDS	5 ROUNDS	5 MINUTES (approximately)	

WARM-UP

The warm-up begins with modified box breathing. The goal is to center the mind, balance our emotional state, lower stress hormones, and decrease anxiety. Equal ratio breathing works to calm the mind, balance our autonomic nervous system, and promote the *sattva guna.* Stress and anxiety can significantly inhibit our ability to focus and retain new memories, which is one reason it is so challenging to study for an important test, prepare for a significant presentation, or remember the details of an argument. We might think that we remember an argument clearly, but every heated discussion I've had with a partner yielded two very different recollections when we revisited the debate. We also remember emotions much stronger than we remember facts, so if we are in an emotional state, we are more likely to clearly recall how we felt rather than the information we were trying to absorb or the factual happenings of an event.

This breath practice increases nitric oxide production and absorption, which helps smooth our emotional state as well as increase our ability to concentrate and learn. The practice begins with a relatively easy equal breath ratio of 5:5:5:5 and maintains this ratio through the five-minute duration of the warm-up. *Bhramari pranayama* (see pages 144 to 147) is added during the exhalation, which increases the cultivation of nitric oxide by fifteen-fold. The five-second outer retention allows nitric oxide to build up even more before taking the next inhalation, which carries the nitric oxide into the lungs and throughout the bloodstream to be delivered to the brain and body tissues. You will continue to use this extended exhalation technique utilizing the *bhramari* breath in the vitalizing component and cool-down in order to fully capitalize on the powerful effects of nitric oxide.

HEAT-BUILDING

The heat-building component intends to increase our energy levels to heighten our awareness, sharpen our focus, and create more mental clarity by invigorating the mind and body. The practice begins with *bhastrika* breath (see pages 126 to 128) to quickly stimulate the sympathetic nervous system and increase *rajas* energy. The *rajas guna* is the energetic quality that provides the drive to achieve our goals and maintains our motivation to see them to completion. The sympathetic nervous system is responsible for alertness. When we activate the sympathetic response, we can shut out distractions and focus on the task at hand. When we play sports or do anything competitive, we have an extremely high sense of awareness and focus, which is a result of the activation of the sympathetic response.

Bhastrika also quickly expels carbon dioxide and increases blood pH, constricting the blood vessels and decreasing the amount of oxygen available to the brain, which in this case is an unwanted effect not conducive to learning. To balance the adverse effects of this practice, we add an outer retention using *uddiyana bandha* (see pages 101 and 102). The outer retention rapidly restores carbon dioxide levels and normalizes blood pH. *Uddiyana bandha* is related to our third *chakra,* which governs willpower and mental vigor, and maintains our *rajasic* energy while stabilizing our sympathetic response. Essentially, it's like drinking a few large cups of coffee and feeling extra alert, but without getting the jittery side effects.

The heat-building component begins with thirty seconds of *bhastrika pranayama,* where you pump the belly like a bellows at a rate of one to two breaths per second, followed by a deep inhalation and a complete exhalation. On the exhalation, tuck your chin and engage *jalandhara bandha* (see pages 102 and 103) and then *uddiyana bandha* by pulling the low belly in toward the spine. Hold outer retention for fifteen seconds. Repeat for six breath cycles, or approximately five minutes.

VITALIZING

The vitalizing component uses an unequal breath ratio combined with *bhramari* breath with the primary intention of increasing the volume and intake of nitric oxide. The humming vibration from *bhramari* stimulates the production and gas exchange of nitric oxide in the paranasal sinuses. Begin the breath practice with a slow ten-second inhalation that is as soft and smooth as possible, similar to how you would smell a perfume. You usually wouldn't take a fast, deep inhalation when smelling a fragrance; more likely, you would inhale slowly and gently to allow the scent to pass over your smell receptors. Breathing in slowly and softly increases the amount of nitric oxide in the nasal cavity and paranasal sinuses.

The inhalation is followed by a twenty-second inner retention. The longer retention gives the lungs more time to absorb nitric oxide and increases carbon dioxide levels, which expands the blood vessels and delivers more oxygen to the brain. Nitric oxide also increases the uptake of oxygen by 10 to 20 percent. If the inner retention feels too challenging to maintain, or if you feel like you need to exhale quickly, then shorten the retention. Physiologically, it is more beneficial for the goal of this practice to maintain slow, smooth inhalations and exhalations than it is to hold longer *kumbhakas.*

After the inner retention, you move into the most important component of this breath practice: the *bhramari* exhalation, which is ten seconds long to match the inhalation. The slow exhalation with *bhramari* breath creates nitric oxide as well as energetically moves you into a *sattvic* state. The primary quality of *sattva* is balance and harmony in the present moment. Most distracting thoughts take you out of the present moment and into irrelevant stories that can disturb your concentration. This *sattvic* aspect of the breath is a powerful component to help you maintain focus and attention. When you exhale with the humming "om" sound, try to push the vibration upward into the nasal cavity and raise the frequency of the sound. Higher resonance creates more vibration and increases nitric oxide levels. After the exhalation, pause for a short five-second outer retention to allow a little time for nitric oxide to build up in the nasal cavity. Repeat this breath cycle for six to twelve rounds, or five to ten minutes.

COOL-DOWN

The cool-down uses modified alternate nostril breathing to balance the mind and harness the full potential of the logical and imaginative aspects of the self. The brain has two hemispheres: the left side is linked to logic, numbers, shapes, and analysis, while the right side is connected to imagination, rhythm, language, and color. It was once thought that the right side was linked to creativity, but we know now that we use the full capacity of the brain to create. The more balanced the mind is, the faster we can generate thoughts and express ideas. When we increase thought fluency, creativity flows from us naturally. *Nadi shodhana* (see pages 132 to 136) uses touch, intention, and visualization to influence both hemispheres of the brain to work together. *Nadi shodhana* has a natural calming effect. You want to focus on a balanced respiration to maintain the *sattvic* energy that you have cultivated throughout the practice while sustaining the other benefits discussed in the vitalizing component. Much of the intention of the vitalizing component is continued through the cool-down, which adds *bhramari* to the exhalation and a short *bahya kumbhaka.*

Begin the practice by holding the two *mudras* associated with *nadi shodhana: jnana mudra* (the wisdom *mudra*) with the left hand and *Vishnu mudra* (the balancing *mudra*) with the right hand. The inhalation always starts through the left nostril because it represents the *ida* channel and the quality of receptivity. Slowly inhale for ten seconds through the left nostril, and then exhale through the right nostril for ten seconds using the *bhramari* technique. Hold outer retention for five seconds. If you want to increase the energy of the practice, you can add on *uddiyana bandha* during the retention. Inhale for ten seconds through the right nostril, exhale with *bhramari pranayama* out the left nostril, and hold for ten seconds.

The left side of the body is linked to the right hemisphere of the brain and vice versa. When breathing through the left nostril, visualize energy traveling up and down the left side of your body and stimulating the right hemisphere of your brain. Switch to the right side of the body and the left hemisphere of the brain when breathing through the right nostril. Continue the cool-down exercise for approximately five minutes, or five or six breath cycles.

ATHLETIC PERFORMANCE

This sequence uses a series of challenging breathing techniques and long breath-holds to lower oxygen availability and increase oxygen demand, simulating high-altitude training (see pages 36 and 37). These breath practices increase cardiorespiratory fitness, strengthen the respiratory muscles, improve VO_2 max, expand vital capacity, and improve overall athletic performance.

Movement and fitness played a massive role in my life from an early age. As a young child, I always wanted to be big and strong. Some of my earliest memories involve working out in my bedroom with a set of three-pound concrete weights to a Hulkamania exercise poster. Maybe it was those early memories that inspired me to get into collegiate and freestyle wrestling, or maybe it was the fact that I was very small for my age but also freakishly strong for my size, and wrestling is a sport that has weight classes, making it easier for smaller athletes to compete. I began wrestling at twelve years old and continued through high school. At eighteen, after joining the Marine Corps, I tried out and made it onto the All-Marine wrestling team, which was an amazing opportunity to continue wrestling and compete at an elite level. During my time on the team, I competed throughout the United States and trained for the 2004 Olympics in Athens. Unfortunately, that dream was cut short in 2003 when I was deployed to Iraq.

A wrestling match lasts only six minutes, but it is probably the most physically demanding six minutes of any sport. During the four years I wrestled for the Marine Corps, my daily regimen consisted of one hour of running, two hours of weight training, and three hours of wrestling practice, which included cardio exercises. Most high-level wrestling matches come down to who has more stamina; while technique and strength are extremely important, you have to be able to outlast your opponent. I remember gasping for air, barely able to breathe enough to supply the amount of oxygen my body needed to meet the intense demand I was putting on it. I recall my muscles burning from high levels of carbon dioxide, my arms and legs nearly immobile, locked up with an opponent who was equally exhausted and struggling. Despite all the training for my wrestling bouts, I never trained how to breathe effectively and efficiently or improve my athletic stamina with breathing, even though winning or losing often comes down to cardiorespiratory endurance.

Most athletes who push themselves to the limit are almost always breathing fast and heavy through an open mouth. This open-mouth breathing is natural because our normal respiratory demand is nowhere near the demand we place on our bodies when we exercise. Even light jogging or walking up a few stairs can increase our need for oxygen to the point where we are huffing for air.

The first time I was instructed to always breathe through my nose was when I started practicing yoga. I can't think of any other physical activity or sport where this is encouraged; however, many athletes now understand the amazing benefits of training while nasal breathing. With yoga, the breath takes precedence over physical movement. If we lose the breath, we stop holding the pose and return to calm nasal breathing and regain control over our breath before resuming the physical practice. Most people understand cardio fitness as having to do with the heart, so we train to get the heart rate up quickly, sustain it, and then recover to our resting heart rate quickly. However, it's not just cardio fitness but cardio*respiratory* fitness, meaning it has to do with the heart *and* the breath. I wish I could go back and teach my younger self how to breathe to improve my athletic performance.

Yoga is not as demanding as most athletic sports, and maybe that's why it is so much easier to breathe through the nose while practicing. However, yoga can be very challenging, and I have noticed that newer practitioners continually resort to mouth breathing as soon as their cardiac demand increases. Nasal breathing while exerting energy takes practice and conditioning. Nasal breathing alone will not increase athletic performance; however, training while nasal breathing will significantly improve athletic performance. Ideally, we want to increase the amount of oxygen we can utilize and deliver throughout the body, also known as VO_2 max. Increasing VO_2 max increases endurance, stamina, and cardiovascular health. For the past several years, I have focused on training while nasal breathing, and whether I am doing yoga, high-intensity workouts, or handstand training, I remain highly aware of how I am breathing. When I practice long handstand holds, I hold water in my mouth to prevent myself from mouth breathing when things start to get challenging.

We can increase our VO_2 max, improve our cardiorespiratory fitness, strengthen our lungs, expand our vital capacity, and improve our athletic performance just by doing breathing exercises. When we are aiming to improve our fitness and athletic performance with breathing, we want to focus on a few particular areas. One is lung capacity. Think of the lungs as the body's gas tank. Larger lungs have more room to hold air and exchange gases to fuel the body. It is debatable whether lung tissue can stretch; most physiologists say that it's not possible. However, it has been shown that lung capacity can be increased; this can be the result of expanding the chest, strengthening our ability to utilize our lungs, or possibly stretching the lungs themselves. For example, earlier I talked about freediver Stig Severinsen, who increased his lung capacity to 14 liters—9 liters more than the average adult.

We also want to increase the strength of our respiratory muscles, especially the diaphragm. If the diaphragm fatigues, then our breathing becomes more labored and less efficient and requires more energy. This is the same with any untrained or unconditioned muscle. Using excess energy to breathe exhausts the skeletal muscles much faster because less oxygen is available to them.

Oxygen is delivered to the body via red blood cells. To increase oxygen delivery, which in turn increases athletic performance and endurance, we need to increase the oxygen saturation of the red blood cells, carried by the hemoglobin, and increase the percentage of red blood cells in the blood, also known as the hematocrit. Our primary means of increasing hematocrit is to boost oxygen demand while lowering oxygen availability. Most of what I talked about in regard to physical training while nasal breathing results in reduced oxygen availability. The body has to adapt by increasing the number of red blood cells, either by splenic contraction, where the spleen releases its store of red blood cells—a short-term solution—or by creating more red blood cells to meet the needs of the body. To achieve this with breathing, we need to decrease our blood oxygen saturation, which is the same as reducing oxygen availability. The most effective way to do so is breath retention, specifically outer retention, or *bahya kumbhaka.* The longer we hold the breath, the less oxygen is available, and the greater the oxygen demand. To be able to hold the breath for an extended time, we need to increase our hematocrit and our tolerance to high levels of carbon dioxide. We also want to increase our vital capacity, which enables us to hold more oxygen in our lungs. When we practice breath-holding, the body senses the lower oxygen saturation, and the kidneys release a hormone called erythropoietin (EPO) that stimulates the production of red blood cells formed in the bone marrow. Outer retention *(bahya kumbhaka)* is more efficient than inner retention *(antara kumbhaka)* because, during outer retention, the decreased air volume means that less oxygen is available for uptake, and carbon dioxide levels rise much faster. However, when we combine outer and inner retention in succession, we can lengthen our efforts to increase oxygen demand and build carbon dioxide tolerance. Inner retention is more approachable for most people beginning to practice breath-holding, and it can be a great way to slowly prepare the mind and body for the more challenging outer retention.

When building up carbon dioxide tolerance, you are going to experience the feeling of breath hunger. Breath hunger can be intense and uncomfortable, especially if you haven't experienced it before. Often breath hunger causes involuntary contractions of the diaphragm, an intense sensation to breathe, and an increase in body temperature. In the beginning, holding the breath while experiencing breath hunger can be challenging. If you have ever fasted, you know that the first day is usually when you experience the most intense hunger pains, which typically subside or get easier to handle as the fast progresses. Breath hunger is similar and gets much easier the more you practice.

Of all the breath sequences that I practice, the sequences that have to do with increasing athletic performance and long breath-holds are my favorite, maybe because I enjoy challenges or because I see so much improvement when I practice them. If you want to increase your athletic endurance or lengthen your breath retention, then I suggest doing this sequence or one you create that is similar to it at least once per week. If you're looking for greater results, then you would want to do this sequence daily, and modify it by increasing hold times when it starts to lose its challenge. This sequence is the most demanding and strenuous in the book. If the retentions are too long, feel free to shorten the duration of the holds. After a short time, you will be able to do these exercises with relative ease.

ATHLETIC PERFORMANCE BREATH SEQUENCE
25–30+ MINUTES

WARM-UP	**LUNG EXPANSION EXERCISE** Maximum inhalation, hold 10 seconds Small expansion inhalation, hold 10 seconds Small expansion inhalation, hold 10 seconds Open mouth exhalation	15 ROUNDS	5 MINUTES (approximately)
HEAT-BUILDING	**BHASTRIKA 1 MINUTE** OUTER RETENTION 30 SECONDS FULL INHALATION INNER RETENTION 1 MINUTE	3 ROUNDS	8 MINUTES (approximately)
VITALIZING	**BREATH RETENTION SEQUENCE** 3 FULL RESPIRATIONS OUTER RETENTION 20 SECONDS INNER RETENTION 40 SECONDS	5 ROUNDS	6 MINUTES
COOL-DOWN	**MAXIMUM RETENTION SEQUENCE** 10 FULL RESPIRATIONS MAXIMUM INNER RETENTION	3–5 ROUNDS	5+ MINUTES

WARM-UP

The warm-up is called the lung expansion exercise and is different from any of the techniques or practices mentioned so far. The primary intention is to expand the lungs and stretch the respiratory muscles.

This exercise is similar to a breathing technique called lung packing. Many freedivers, both novice and elite, practice lung packing to expand their vital capacity and increase their oxygen reserves. They inhale as much air as possible before diving, completely filling the lungs and then "packing" in more air with small inhalations, sometimes up to sixty packs. Overpacking can be very dangerous, and I don't recommend trying lung packing without an experienced freediving coach to guide you.

The lung expansion exercise is a much gentler practice that involves taking a full inhalation and holding it for ten seconds to allow the chest and lungs to expand for a short time, similar to holding a stretch before going deeper. While maintaining the inner retention, take another very small nasal inhalation and hold for ten more seconds. Repeat this process once more, for a total of two extra lung expansion inhalations in addition to the initial inhalation, and three ten-second inner retentions. After the third retention, exhale out of the mouth and empty the lungs. Each ten-second hold gives time for the lungs to expand, the air to settle, and the intercostal muscles to stretch. This succession of short inner retentions also gradually accustoms the body to rising carbon dioxide levels and builds up your carbon dioxide tolerance. The inhalations and expansion breaths should not be painful. You might experience slight discomfort, just like you would when stretching any other muscle. Repeat this exercise ten times.

Note: Overdoing the lung expansion exercise or any other lung packing exercise by either inhaling to the point of pain or overpacking the lungs is potentially harmful and may result in pulmonary barotrauma.

HEAT-BUILDING

The heat-building component has three parts that work to strengthen the respiratory muscles and train breath retention. It starts with a one-minute *bhastrika pranayama.* As you do this practice, put even more focus on moving your stomach in and out to strengthen your core muscles and diaphragm. As you perform the *bhastrika* breath, you are expelling a large amount of carbon dioxide and becoming very alkaline. After one minute of bellows breath, exhale fully and hold outer retention for thirty seconds, followed by a full inhalation and a one-minute inner retention. Because of the carbon dioxide deficiency created from the *bhastrika* practice, both the inner and outer retentions should be relatively easy, especially compared to how challenging the retentions would be without doing this controlled hyperventilation first. The carbon dioxide deficiency also provides more time in the breath-hold to lower blood oxygen saturation but less time to build up carbon dioxide tolerance. However, the main objective of the heat-building component is to strengthen the respiratory muscles. If the breath retentions are too challenging in the beginning, shorten them to a more manageable duration. After one minute of *antara kumbhaka,* take a complete exhalation and repeat the breath cycle two more times, starting with the *bhastrika* breath.

VITALIZING

The vitalizing component switches the focus to the breath retention and the increase of carbon dioxide tolerance to lower oxygen availability and increase oxygen demand. The breath-holds in this component are one-third the length of the holds in the heat-building component; however, because you are not initiating the retention with *bhastrika,* this practice can be slightly more challenging. It begins with three regular nasal breaths followed by a full exhalation and a twenty-second outer retention. After the outer retention, take a single inhalation and hold the breath for forty more seconds. In the heat-building component, you were continuously breathing off large amounts of carbon dioxide, which made the subsequent breath-holds less challenging. The vitalizing practice gives you an insufficient number of respirations to regulate your carbon dioxide levels, so each breath retention becomes more difficult. Ideally, you want to be experiencing a slight amount of breath hunger toward the end. If the holds are too short or too long, adjust them until the final round pushes you to the point where you feel some breath hunger but are not pushed to your breath-holding limit. Repeat for five breath cycles.

COOL-DOWN

The cool-down pushes you to your breath-holding edge. It begins with ten full, deep nasal inhalations and either an open mouth or a nasal exhalation. An open mouth exhalation can make it easier to breathe off more carbon dioxide quicker. These breaths shouldn't feel like hyperventilation even though they technically are; the deep, uninterrupted breaths enable you to breathe off a considerable amount of carbon dioxide before beginning the breath-hold. After ten respirations, take a full, deep breath and hold inner retention for as long as possible. You want to experience some breath hunger here; as you practice and get more accustomed to the sensation, you can remain in this phase for longer and feel more comfortable. Once you reach your limit of the first breath, exhale and repeat the process two more times, beginning again with ten deep respirations. When you start practicing these retentions, aim for two minutes or slightly longer. Over time, you'll be able to increase the duration to four minutes or longer. For some people, each subsequent retention is more difficult than the last. For me, my third hold is usually a minute or more longer than my first hold. This has to do with the splenic contraction releasing more red blood cells into circulation through the course of the sequence. The cool-down is my favorite part of this practice because I can see my personal growth from my training and effort.

I suggest that you do this breath sequence with a timer and keep track of your results. Also, be aware that lengths of your breath retentions will fluctuate; some days they will be longer than others. Your performance will vary up and down, but it will slowly increase over time—just not overnight. I find it helpful to keep track of other factors that affect my breath retention, such as sleep, diet, and stress, and determine what is affecting me the most so I can improve those areas of my life.

INCREASED METABOLISM AND WEIGHT LOSS

This breath sequence, if done regularly, can help boost metabolism, aid in weight loss, decrease appetite, reduce stress hormones that lead to over-eating, and tone and firm the belly. The practice involves a series of rapid breathing and core engagement exercises balanced by stress-lowering breath retention practices.

The first thing that most people think about when metabolism is mentioned is weight loss. And that's probably for good reason, since most of us are concerned with our weight, and that includes slender and fit people. Healthy people are generally concerned with their weight, which is likely a part of their motivation to stay in shape. Maintaining a healthy diet and an active lifestyle with adequate exercise takes effort. However, the amount of work it takes is not equal for everyone. Some of us are born with faster metabolisms and are naturally skinny because of our genetics, while others have to work hard to lose every ounce of fat.

I have always cared about how much fat I have on my body. When I was younger, I could eat anything and never gain weight. That was partly because of how active I was and partly because of my extremely fast metabolism. Both of my parents were skinny, and I grew up obsessed with fitness. Now that I'm getting older, I have noticed my metabolism slowing down, and I need to pay more attention to how much I eat, the quality of my food, and how much I move.

No matter which diet we choose, how we like to exercise, or how slow or fast our metabolism is, losing weight comes down to burning more calories than we take in. Of course, diet, exercise, and metabolism all directly affect the weight-loss equation. The quality of calories makes a huge difference as well. A 300-calorie slice of pizza is not equivalent to a 300-calorie salad.

Without spending too much time discussing the pros and cons of different diets, my recommendation when it comes to nutrition is to eat foods that make you feel good—and by "feel good," I don't mean how that chocolate bar helps when you feel sad, but food that gives you energy and doesn't make you feel sick, slow, or heavy after you eat. If you are unsure of what those foods are, start by cutting out any food that has a commercial. If someone needs to persuade you to eat it, it's probably not healthy for you. If you look at the label and don't recognize everything listed, then your body probably won't recognize it as food. When you go grocery shopping, the real food is generally around the perimeter of the store, and the stuff to avoid is usually down the aisles. It is vital to eat nutrient-dense foods; we are what we eat, and the foods we eat can speed up or slow down our metabolism.

My expertise is primarily in health and fitness. When it comes to helping people exercise to lose weight, my advice is simple: move more than you're already doing. It really doesn't matter what you do as long as you move more than you eat. Start with easy exercises. Yoga is great for providing movements that anyone can do and catering to all fitness levels. When you get to a place where you can put more effort into your exercise, then high-intensity, fast-recovery exercises will burn the most calories in the least amount of time. High-intensity exercises also stimulate our metabolism.

Most people know that metabolism has something to do with burning calories for fuel, losing weight, or increasing energy levels, but there is so much more to it than that. Metabolism encompasses the controlled chemical reactions that happen inside our cells, which take things like food and air from the environment, break them down into various molecules, and transform them into energy and replacement parts for the cells. Cellular metabolism consists of hundreds of chemical reactions, either catabolic, which break molecules apart, or anabolic, which join molecules together to create new molecules. Our bodies need nutrients to build, maintain, and repair themselves. When we eat, our bodies break down food into fats, sugars, and amino acids, which are then converted and utilized, turned into energy, or expelled as waste. All fats and sugars are composed solely of molecular compounds that are made up of carbon, hydrogen, and oxygen. Amino acids, which make up the various proteins, are also composed of carbon, hydrogen, and oxygen, along with nitrogen and sulfur.

I said that to lose weight, we need to burn more calories than we take in. But where do those calories go? The first law of thermodynamics, as quoted by Einstein, states, "Energy cannot be created nor destroyed; it can only be transferred or changed from one form to another." We can't just burn energy, and then it goes away. So what happens to the calories we burn? Where does the fat go? The answer is that we exhale most of it as carbon dioxide. As discussed in the section on cellular respiration (see pages 16 and 17), which also has to do with metabolism, the body takes glucose and oxygen and converts them to energy, which the cells use to drive anabolic reactions; water and carbon dioxide are exhaled. Water, or H_2O, is made up of two hydrogen atoms and one oxygen atom. Carbon dioxide, or CO_2, is composed of one carbon atom and two oxygen atoms. Both water and carbon dioxide are made from the same building blocks as sugars and fats. When we burn fat, the fat is broken down and converted to water and carbon dioxide, which again we exhale. Proteins are the same, except that the extra nitrogens and sulfurs are converted to urea and sulfates, which are expelled through the urine and feces.

If we lose 10 kilograms (22 pounds) of fat, 8.4 kilograms (18.5 pounds) is converted to carbon dioxide and exhaled and 1.6 kilograms (3.5 pounds) is converted to water, which is sweated out, urinated or defecated out, or exhaled.[4] When we lose weight, anything we burn off has to be expelled through breathing. One reason high-intensity training and cardio exercise are so effective for weight loss is that they increase our respiratory rate. Therefore, we are able to expel more of the carbon that is responsible for those extra pounds.

Of course, we shouldn't just start hyperventilating to lose weight. We still need to regulate the autonomic nervous system and keep our blood pH balanced. Also, retaining carbon dioxide with breath-holding does not lead to weight gain. Only plants can convert carbon dioxide to fats, sugars, and proteins, which is why plants give off oxygen while human beings exhale carbon dioxide.

The goal is to boost metabolism, burn calories, and convert fat and sugar to carbon dioxide to be exhaled. We also want to use the breath to reduce stress hormones that lead to over-eating and regulate blood pH to help decrease appetite and promote healthier food cravings. We first need to stimulate the sympathetic nervous system to increase our heart and respiratory rates, which will burn more calories and expel the converted fats and sugars as carbon dioxide. Then we need to work into longer holds that create a more parasympathetic tone and lower blood pH.

This breath sequence progresses through a significant energetic wave with several rapid breathing exercises that build quickly to ramp up our energy, and then the vitalizing and cool-down components bring it back down so that we leave the practice in a calm and centered state. What we do after the practice is just as important as what we do during the practice. If the breath sequence focused only on practices that boost metabolism, then chances are, the rapid breathing exercises would lead to high-calorie food cravings. Therefore, we want to end the breath sequence with exercises that increase carbon dioxide to help curb our appetite and food cravings.

This breath sequence is the most beneficial if practiced after a workout, when the heart rate is already increased. We can further boost the metabolic rate and weight loss with the rapid breathing exercises and then follow with the regulating *kumbhaka* practices.

METABOLISM AND WEIGHT LOSS BREATH SEQUENCE
25–27 MINUTES

1:1:1 | INHALATION:INNER RETENTION:EXHALATION   1:1:1:1 | INHALATION:INNER RETENTION:EXHALATION:OUTER RETENTION

WARM-UP	**BREATH OF FIRE 1 MINUTE** *AGNISAR* 20 REPS (ABDOMINAL CONTRACTIONS)	5 ROUNDS	6 MINUTES (approximately)
HEAT-BUILDING 1	**KAPALABHATI 30 SECONDS** *UDDIYANA BANDHA* 10 SECONDS INNER RETENTION 20 SECONDS	5 ROUNDS	5 MINUTES (approximately)
HEAT-BUILDING 2	**BHASTRIKA 10 SECONDS** INNER RETENTION 10 SECONDS *BHASTRIKA* 10 SECONDS OUTER RETENTION 20 SECONDS	6 ROUNDS	5 MINUTES (approximately)
VITALIZING	*VISHAMA VRITTI* 5:10:10:5 *VISHAMA VRITTI* 5:20:10:5 *VISHAMA VRITTI* 5:30:10:5	3 ROUNDS 3 ROUNDS 3 ROUNDS	6 MINUTES (approximately)
COOL-DOWN	*VISHAMA VRITTI* 10:20:10 *SAMA VRITTI* 10:10	5 ROUNDS 5 ROUNDS	5 MINUTES (approximately)

WARM-UP

The warm-up begins with the breath of fire *pranayama* to build internal heat, stimulate the sympathetic nervous system, and increase your respiratory rate. As you progress with this fast breathing exercise, you want to gradually decrease your carbon dioxide levels to prepare for the *agnisar* exercise that follows. After one minute of breath of fire, take one full inhalation and a complete exhalation. While holding the exhalation, begin twenty repetitions of *agnisar,* contracting the stomach and pulling the navel toward the spine as though you are trying to hollow out the belly by sucking in without actually inhaling. While still holding the breath, release and expand the abdomen by completely relaxing the core muscles. Repeat the pumping action of sucking in and contracting the belly and then releasing the stomach.

This exercise is challenging because it involves outer retention. If twenty repetitions is too challenging, do as many as you can. Likewise, if twenty repetitions feels too easy, feel free to add more. The practice increases the strength and endurance of the abdominal muscles, especially the deeper core muscles, accessory breathing muscles, and diaphragm. Strengthening the respiratory muscles and diaphragm improves respiratory function and boosts your resting metabolic rate. After a round of *agnisar,* take an intermediate respiration and continue with another cycle of breath of fire. Each round consists of one minute of breath of fire and twenty repetitions of *agnisar.* Move through this breath cycle five times.

HEAT-BUILDING

The heat-building component continues the intention of the warm-up exercise. Through the first half of this practice, you are trying to increase your respirations to expel as much carbon dioxide as possible, strengthen your core muscles, and increase your heart rate and cardiorespiratory endurance, which will also increase your metabolic rate.

The first part of the heat-building component begins with thirty seconds of *kapalabhati pranayama. Kapalabhati* is slightly more challenging to maintain than breath of fire and requires more abdominal strength and movement. The core muscles needed to do this practice adequately should already be warmed up from the five rounds of *agnisar.* After thirty seconds of *kapalabhati,* take a full inhalation and a complete exhalation, tuck the chin and engage *jalandhara bandha* (throat lock; see pages 102 and 103), lift *uddiyana bandha* (abdominal lock; see page 101) by pulling the navel toward the spine, and hold for ten seconds. Follow the outer retention with a full inhalation and a twenty-second inner retention. *Uddiyana bandha* works similarly to *agnisar* but in a more static way. The difference is like doing push-ups versus holding a plank position. The breath retention in this practice is to regulate over-breathing and becoming too alkaline. If you were to practice all these rapid breathing exercises without the breath-holds, you would become light-headed and dizzy. Repeat this breath cycle for five rounds before moving on.

The second part of the heat-building component increases the intensity of the rapid breathing and begins to energetically make the switch to the vitalizing component by promoting more parasympathetic tone with the longer retentions in relation to the time spent in fast breathing. It begins with a powerful *bhastrika* exercise for ten seconds while rapidly pumping the belly in and out. This exercise is followed by a ten-second inner retention and then returns to ten more seconds of *bhastrika,* followed by twenty seconds of outer retention. When you finish the outer retention, that's one breath cycle. Repeat this cycle six times, or for about five minutes. This second part of the heat-building component switches quickly between a sympathetic-stimulating exercise and a parasympathetic-stimulating exercise. You should start to feel more energetic balance and a calming effect with the twenty-second outer retentions as they slowly reduce sympathetic tone and reestablish your normal carbon dioxide levels.

VITALIZING

The vitalizing component switches gears as the sequence moves from the intention of increasing energy and boosting metabolism to the secondary intention of reducing stress hormones that can lead to stress eating, decreasing appetite, and influencing blood pH to stimulate healthy cravings. The sequence progresses through variations of *vishama vritti* where the breath retentions gradually increase in length and difficulty to build up carbon dioxide levels and stimulate the parasympathetic nervous system. It starts with three rounds of 5:10:10:5, followed by three rounds of 5:20:10:5, and finishes with three rounds of 5:30:10:5. The slower breath rate and longer retentions make the blood pH slightly more acidic. The acidic pH signals the body to regulate the blood to become more alkaline. The body does so through faster breathing, which you consciously control, and by craving alkaline-forming foods, such as vegetables and fruits. Increasing blood pH also works to suppress appetite.

COOL-DOWN

The cool-down continues the intention of the vitalizing component while creating a calmer and more peaceful state with an easier retention practice. It begins with five rounds of 10:20:10, leaving out the outer retention and focusing more on a balanced inhalation and exhalation. It concludes with five rounds of 10:10 *sama vritti pranayama.* The last five *sama vritti* breaths should be only as deep as necessary. You want to finish the practice feeling calm and relaxed, with the nervous system in a perfect state of balance.

LIBIDO AND SEXUAL AROUSAL

This tantric-style breath sequence is designed to cultivate sexual appetite, manifest our intimate desires, and help us form a deep connection with our partner through the exchange of sexual energy. We move through breathing exercises that help regulate the nervous system and decrease stress hormones that lower testosterone availability. We also use breathing practices that increase arousal and sensitivity and lead to more intense orgasms.

Years ago, one of my teachers explained to me the difference between love and attachment. *Attachment,* she said, is about wanting someone to make us happy. *Love* is about wishing happiness for someone else. Unfortunately, most of us confuse the need for others to make us happy with love. Another term often conflated with attachment is *connection.* In yoga, many practitioners both question and struggle to fully understand the philosophy of non-attachment. Why wouldn't we want to be attached to the people we love?

This returns to substituting attachment for love. When we lose a loved one, we feel pain. Pain comes from the separation we feel from the loss of that person. Connection is the root of love, and separation is the cause of all suffering. When we are attached to something or someone, the attachment exists because that person or thing makes us happy. In turn, we want the people and things to which we are attached to remain unchanged so that they will continue to be a source of happiness in our lives. Unfortunately, nothing stays the same, so when we lose what we identify as our source of happiness, that separation creates suffering. When we lose someone we love, whether it's by way of death or the end of a relationship, we immediately feel that separation and the accompanying suffering. The pain eventually fades because we realize we don't need that person to make us happy. Instead, we only feel our connection and love for that person. The pain diminishes because the attachment was an illusion, but the love remains because our connection is real. Because we are all connected, time, distance, and even death cannot separate us. I'm not saying attachments are wrong or that we shouldn't be attached to the people we love. To be attached is human—and so is suffering. However, understanding the difference between connection and attachment can help us through times when loss creates pain.

There are many ways to express love and show affection. At the center of intimacy are love and connection. We often use sex to feel a more profound sense of connection with each other. Physically, it is the closest we can be to someone. Emotionally, intimacy creates a space that allows us to be open and vulnerable to each other. When the sex is good, the emotions and feelings are that much more intense, and we feel even more unified. The problem arises when we confuse sex for connection or use sex to try to feel connected when the connection isn't there. Often, our expectations of what sex *should be* creates sexual dysfunction. We think we need to look or perform a certain way and have sex so many times a week (or day) to be adequate lovers. The more pressure we put on sex, the worse it can be. If intimacy is about connection, then to connect genuinely to our partner, we need to be connected to ourselves.

Healthy relationships start with love, appreciation, and acceptance. If this is the foundation of your relationship, then you and your partner will grow, change, and develop in a healthy way that creates an even deeper connection. But if you think your partner is unappealing, inadequate, and in need of change, then your relationship will likely be dysfunctional and unhealthy, and your sex life will suffer as a result.

Our relationships with our bodies are no different. If you think your body is disgusting and inadequate, then it is not your body that needs to change but your relationship to it. We care for the things we love, not view them with disgust. You can't change your body and expect that your view of it will change. You must first change how you see yourself, how you love yourself, and even how you see yourself as being desirable. Affirmations such as "I love myself and my body!" are more powerful than all the sit-ups in the world. Ultimately, when you love yourself, you learn how to take care of yourself, and then you learn how to feel good about yourself. Feeling good about yourself and feeling confident in your appearance are as essential to sexual function as being attracted to your partner.

There are several possible reasons for low libido or sex drive. It could have to do with a dysfunctional or stale relationship. It could stem from being overly busy and too exhausted at the end of the day, too much stress at work, a lack of desire, or an underlying medical condition. If it is an issue with the relationship, usually the sex will suffer, so to improve our libido, we need to work on the connection with our partner. Of course, this is an oversimplification of something very complicated, but I do believe that most difficulties with intimacy can be solved through self-exploration, honesty, transparency, and, most of all, good communication. Great sex can improve a relationship and deepen the connection, but sex will not fix a bad relationship.

And, unfortunately, bad or infrequent sex and a lack of sexual intimacy can severely harm a relationship. Of course, every relationship is different, and some people place more value on sex than others. Everyone has a different sex drive, different turn-ons, and different sexual desires. We shouldn't compare ourselves to what we think is normal because there is no "normal." We need to understand and be open to our partner's needs and desires as well as our own and be willing to compromise, but of course, this can only happen through clear and honest communication.

Even people in healthy intimate relationships struggle with their sex life or lack thereof. It can be easy to become complacent when it comes to sex, especially in a long-term relationship in which sex has become routine or has lost its importance. When we don't place value on sex, it's easy to make excuses for why we shouldn't put in the effort. Without a healthy libido, we might choose to sleep or rest instead of having sex. Chronic stress, an overly active mind, an unbalanced nervous system, and hormones are usually the culprits.

We need to manifest our sexual energy, cultivate our intimate desires, and form a deep connection to our partner while exchanging a flow of sexual energy. A lack of intimacy generally comes from a lack of presence. The more we are in the moment with our partner, the deeper we can establish our bond of intimacy. Meditation and *pranayama* are powerful practices to train the mind to be present and less distracted. We can use the breath to alleviate some of the hindrances that suppress libido, such as high stress hormones and an autonomic nervous system imbalance. We can also use the breath to increase sexual energy and improve blood flow to the penis and/or clitoris to increase erectile ability and sex drive.

This breath sequence can be done alone, but it is so much more powerful when it's done with your partner in an intimate setting, where you can cultivate sexual energy, be aroused by listening to your partner's breath, and let your deep connection add to the eroticism. Whether you are doing this practice alone or with your partner, focus your attention around your genitals throughout the practice. With every exhalation, send more sexual energy into the genitals. You can keep your eyes closed and visualize your partner or keep them open and gaze into each other's eyes or at each other's bodies. This breath practice can be a very intimate form of foreplay, and physical touch is encouraged throughout the practice.

LIBIDO AND SEXUAL AROUSAL BREATH SEQUENCE 14–16 MINUTES			
1:1 | INHALATION:EXHALATION	**1:1:1:1 | INHALATION:INNER RETENTION:EXHALATION:OUTER RETENTION**		
WARM-UP	**RAJAS BREATH** (*UJJAYI* INHALATION:SIGH EXHALATION) 5:1 8:1 10:1	5 ROUNDS 5 ROUNDS 5 ROUNDS	2 MINUTES (approximately)
HEAT-BUILDING	**NADI SHODHANA/KAPALABHATI** 30 SECONDS ALTERNATE NOSTRIL BREATHING WITH 3 *KAPALABHATI* BREATHS PER NOSTRIL (R,R,R–L,L,L)	3 ROUNDS	6 MINUTES
VITALIZING	**VISHAMA VRITTI 4:16:8:4** *Ujjayi* on inhalation *Bhramari* on exhalation *Uddiyana bandha* on outer retention	10 ROUNDS	5 MINUTES (approximately)
COOL-DOWN	**SAMA VRITTI 10:10** *Ujjayi* on inhalation *Bhramari* on exhalation	10 ROUNDS	3 MINUTES (approximately)

WARM-UP

The warm-up uses the *rajas* breath to stimulate the sympathetic nervous system and increase *rajas* energy—the energy of passion and play. It is associated with new life and reproduction, and it's this type of energy that ignites our sexual urges. This breath practice uses a longer inhalation with a short, powerful open-mouth sighing exhalation to cultivate *rajasic* energy. It also adds a strong *ujjayi* technique to the inhalation. Both the *ujjayi* inhalation and the sighing exhalation should be audible. These sounds, especially if you are listening to your partner's breath, can be very arousing and have an autonomous sensory meridian response (ASMR) effect, which can be very erotic for some people. The warm-up starts with a five-second *ujjayi* inhalation and sighing exhalation, which you repeat five times. Then lengthen the inhalation to eight seconds, repeating five times, and then to ten seconds, also repeating five times. Feel the energy of each exhalation moving downward and building in your genitals. If the increasing inhalation duration feels too complicated, you can stick with the middle ratio of 8:1 and repeat it for fifteen rounds. It's also not necessary that you do the exact number of rounds. It can be more beneficial to do an intuitive number of rounds. This is true for all the components of this breath sequence.

HEAT-BUILDING

The heat-building component combines *nadi shodhana* and *kapalabhati pranayama* practices with short retentions. *Nadi shodhana* balances *ida* energy, which is the energy of receiving, nurturing, and intuition, with *pingala* energy, which is the energy of power, assertiveness, and giving. All these qualities are necessary for the exchange of sexual energy with a partner.

Add *kapalabhati* by alternating three breaths per nostril, switching back and forth between the left and right sides. It's more important to have strong abdominal contractions on the exhalation than to breathe fast. It is probably better to go a little slower so that you can focus on the energetic cultivation. Do this practice for ten breath cycles, three breaths on the left side and three on the right side equaling one cycle, and then follow the breath with an inner retention for thirty seconds. The breath retention after fast breathing is powerful at releasing stress hormones such as cortisol, which can lower the availability of testosterone. As you hold your breath, bring the sensation into your body so that you can expand your sexual energy. Repeat this heat-building practice three times.

VITALIZING

The vitalizing component brings us more into the parasympathetic nervous system. Sex is one of the few instances in which the sympathetic and parasympathetic nervous systems can be fully active simultaneously. Arousal, sexual stimulation, and erections are functions of the parasympathetic nervous system, while orgasms and ejaculation are functions of the sympathetic nervous system. The goal is to regulate both systems to create balance, but also to highlight the parasympathetic nervous system to feel more relaxed, open, and connected.

This practice utilizes *vishama vritti* to add breath retention, increase carbon dioxide levels, and stimulate the parasympathetic nervous system. You add *ujjayi* to the inhalation to help maintain the passionate *rajasic* energy you cultivated, and you add *bhramari* to the exhalation. The humming from *bhramari* breath increases nitric oxide levels. Nitric oxide opens the blood vessels, which increases blood flow to the genitalia. Men get harder erections, and women get more blood flow to the clitoris, creating more pressure, more sensitivity, and more intense orgasms. This vasodilation in the genitals works similarly to the effects of drugs like Viagra and Cialis that enhance nitric oxide–mediated vasodilation in the erectile tissues.

The vitalizing practice uses the standard *vishama vritti* breath ratio of 1:4:2:1. I suggest starting with 4:16:8:4; if that duration feels challenging, modify it to 3:12:6:3. The breath ratio should be relatively easy, especially if your partner is not used to doing longer breath-holds. If it's too challenging, it can bring you out of the moment, but you want the sequence to be long enough to build up your carbon dioxide levels and stimulate the parasympathetic nervous system. Repeat this practice ten times, or for about five minutes. As you move through this practice, try to match the inhalations and exhalations with your partner's, but keep the breath count silent. By practicing like this, you learn to listen to your partner, to feel their breath and respond to their energy. This in itself is an amazing exercise for nonverbal communication.

COOL-DOWN

The cool-down brings out your sensuality. It uses an equal ratio of 10:10 with a strong *ujjayi* on the inhalation and *bhramari* during the exhalation. Equal ratio breathing regulates the autonomic nervous system, which stimulates the ventral vagal complex and promotes a feeling of safety and freedom. The shared audible breath encourages openness and communication and lowers inhibitions. Both *ujjayi* and *bhramari* continue to affect the mind and body in the ways expressed in the previous exercises. Continue the breath for approximately ten cycles or until you feel you have achieved your goals for the sequence.

POST-WORKOUT RECOVERY

This breath sequence is designed to speed up recovery time after a workout by regulating the autonomic nervous system and increasing parasympathetic tone to help increase cardiorespiratory recovery and improve circulation. These exercises are centered on maintaining slow breathing with intermittent breath retention to build up carbon dioxide and nitric oxide levels that increase cellular oxygenation and aid in muscle recovery.

One of the most powerful aspects of the breath when it comes to recovery is its ability to suppress the sympathetic nervous system and stimulate the parasympathetic response. The parasympathetic nervous system is classically coined the rest-and-digest or rest-and-recovery system. It is responsible for slowing our heart and respiratory rates, opening up our blood vessels to increase blood flow, and lowering blood pressure to recover the spent energy used while in a sympathetic state.

When we do any type of physical activity, whether it's jumping up off the couch to answer the door or running a marathon, our bodies need energy to move our muscles. Obviously, the amount of energy required to run to the door is much less than the amount needed to run a marathon. Also, the body uses different systems to create energy for these activities. The energy to power muscles and cells comes in the form of adenosine triphosphate, or ATP. ATP is the universal fuel for the body. As the body consumes ATP, the ATP molecule loses one phosphate group and releases energy for us to utilize. ATP becomes adenosine diphosphate (ADP), which has two phosphate groups instead of three. For ADP to release more energy, it needs to regain its missing phosphate group and transform back into ATP. We've already discussed how ATP is made through cellular respiration, the process of aerobic glycolysis or the action of converting glucose to ATP using oxygen. (*Aerobic* means "with oxygen," and glycolysis is the process of breaking down sugars using enzymes.)

When we are at rest, the amount of oxygen we need is equal to the amount of oxygen supplied; this is our steady-state, or oxygen homeostasis. As soon as we increase our activity level, exceeding our steady-state, we require more energy (ATP) and oxygen to meet the increased demand. ATP is readily available, but oxygen supply is not. It takes a short time for the sympathetic nervous system to respond and increase the heart and respiratory rates to meet our oxygen needs. This lack of readily available oxygen places us in a state of oxygen deficiency. Luckily, the body has three ways of creating energy, and two of those don't require oxygen to produce ATP. As soon as we move into an oxygen-deficient state, the body starts producing energy anaerobically, meaning without oxygen.

The first way the body creates energy is via the alactacid (without lactic acid) system, sometimes referred to as the ATP PC system because phosphate and creatine, or phosphocreatine, are required to generate ATP. Our muscles readily store phosphocreatine to be immediately converted to energy during intense physical activity. These stores of phosphocreatine quickly run out after eight to twelve seconds, releasing energy and heat as a by-product. It takes the body anywhere from thirty seconds to two minutes to restore the alactacid system so that we can use it again.

After this first system is exhausted, the body switches to the lactic acid system for the bulk of its immediate energy needs. The lactic acid system converts stored sugars (glycogen) to energy without oxygen through a process called anaerobic glycolysis, using several complex chemical reactions. The glycogen breaks down into ATP, hydrogen (H) ions, and pyruvic acid. We can sustain anaerobic activity for approximately thirty seconds to three minutes while our oxygen supply builds up to meet our oxygen demand. Pyruvic acid and hydrogen ions increase the acidity levels in the muscles, leading to muscle fatigue. When oxygen is available, the pyruvic acid is converted to energy via the citric acid cycle (also known as the Krebs cycle). If there is not sufficient oxygen available, then pyruvic acid goes through a process called fermentation and produces lactic acid.[5] However, lactic acid is no longer thought to lead to delayed-onset muscle soreness (DOMS). DOMS is mostly believed to be caused by tiny tears in the muscles from eccentric contractions (increased tension on the total length of the muscle).

Our anaerobic systems are not resistant to fatigue and wear out quickly. Once our oxygen supply increases to meet demand, the body switches to aerobic glycolysis. If we can't raise oxygen supply to reach our oxygen deficit quickly enough because our VO_2 max (the amount of oxygen the body can utilize during exercise) is insufficient, then we won't be able to sustain aerobic activity and we will experience exhaustion. As soon as we can meet the demand for oxygen, the aerobic system becomes our primary source for creating energy by converting sugars and oxygen to ATP and releasing carbon dioxide and water as the by-products. We should be familiar with this third system of aerobic glycolysis by now, since this is the main action of cellular respiration and why we breathe. Aerobic glycolysis runs primarily off of our glycogen (sugar) stores, but once those are used up, the body switches to burning fat. It usually takes about two hours to use up our sugar stores, but once we do, fatigue begins to set in. Converting fat to energy requires significantly more oxygen than sugar and is much more work for the body and cardiorespiratory system. This fatigue is commonly known as "hitting the wall." Recovering our glycogen stores takes twenty-four to forty-eight hours. The more we train and exercise, the quicker we are able to meet our aerobic homeostasis, or the state where oxygen supply meets oxygen demand. We're able to reach this state quicker because we can increase our heart rate and breathing faster, decreasing the amount of time spent in the anaerobic phase, which means less oxygen deficiency and quicker recovery.

After exercising, we move into the final phase, which is often referred to as the afterburn effect but is more accurately termed excess post-exercise oxygen consumption (EPOC). For up to several hours after any strenuous activity, the body continues to use more oxygen than usual. EPOC, or continuation of increased consumption of oxygen, is the beginning of the recovery phase. During EPOC, we continue to burn between 6 and 15 percent of the amount of energy we used during exercise.[6] As we start resting, our bodies are still carrying out many of the functions that were active while we were exercising. Even though we have finished our workout, our sympathetic nervous system remains dominant, and we continue to have elevated levels of epinephrine (adrenaline) and norepinephrine. Our metabolic rate is still increased, and we require more oxygen. Our heart rate and respiratory rate have not returned to normal, and our bodies need to continue using energy to replace the phosphocreatine store and remove any excess lactic acid. EPOC can last for one hour to several hours post-exercise,[7] and while we are in this phase, it is vital to increase our oxygen to speed up our recovery time.

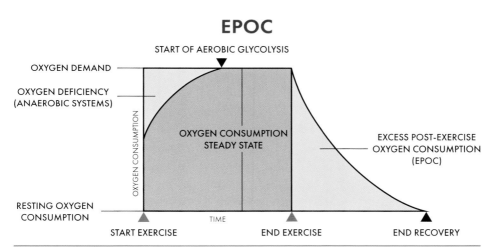

At rest, our oxygen demand meets our oxygen consumption. When we begin physical activity, there is an immediate increase in oxygen demand that isn't met. To compensate, we create energy via our anaerobic (without oxygen) systems. We can sustain anaerobic activity for only a few minutes. Once oxygen demand is met, the body switches its energy production to the aerobic (with oxygen) system. When we finish the activity, we have a recovery period of increased oxygen consumption, called excess post-exercise oxygen consumption (EPOC). During the EPOC phase, the body consumes more oxygen and burns energy, even at rest. Decreasing EPOC time is a sign of improved athletic performance and recovery.

Once we finish exercising and begin the recovery process, we want to quickly shift our autonomic nervous system to stimulate our parasympathetic nervous system. The activation of the parasympathetic nervous system slows our heart rate, opens our blood vessels to increase blood flow, and lowers our adrenaline levels. We can increase the uptake of oxygen into the cells, which will also help decrease lactic acid and increase energy production from pyruvic acid by elevating our carbon dioxide levels with breath retention. We also want to increase our nitric oxide levels. Nitric oxide helps decrease the inflammatory response, speeds up cellular regeneration, and aids in repairing muscle fibers, as well as increases blood flow to remove waste by-products from exercise and increase cellular oxygenation.[8]

Begin this post-workout recovery sequence in a comfortable seated position, adhering to all the guidelines for good breathing posture (see pages 41 and 42), or practice in a reclined recovery position. I recommend that you lie on your back next to a wall, elevate your hips slightly on a small pad or bolster, and extend your legs up the wall or place your feet against the wall, with your knees wide and slightly bent. This position can help reduce stress and fatigue, and it's a great posture that facilitates venous return from the lower extremities and increases circulation.

POST-WORKOUT RECOVERY BREATH SEQUENCE
18–20 MINUTES

	1:x:1:1 | INHALATION:EXHALATION:OUTER RETENTION	1:1:1 | INHALATION:INNER RETENTION:EXHALATION	
WARM-UP	**BHASTRIKA 10 SECONDS** OUTER RETENTION 15 SECONDS INNER RETENTION 30 SECONDS	5 ROUNDS	5 MINUTES (approximately)
HEAT-BUILDING	**VISHAMA VRITTI 5:x:5:10** (inhale for 5 seconds, exhale for 5 seconds, hold outer retention for 10 seconds)	15 ROUNDS	5 MINUTES (approximately)
VITALIZING	**VISHAMA VRITTI 5:20:5 | 5:x:5:20** (inhale for 5 seconds, hold inner retention for 20 seconds, exhale for 5 seconds; inhale for 5 seconds, exhale for 5 seconds, hold outer retention for 20 seconds)	10 ROUNDS	5 MINUTES (approximately)
COOL-DOWN	**SAMA VRITTI 15:15* ➡ 5:5*** *Bhramari on exhalation 15:15 decrease each respiration by 1:1 until finishing at 5:5 (15:15, 14:14, 13:13,...5:5)	1 ROUND	4 MINUTES (approximately)

WARM-UP

The warm-up starts a little differently compared to most of the warm-up practices in this book. You begin faster than you would for most recovery practices with *bhastrika pranayama.* Normally, the *bhastrika* practice would be in the heat-building component. Considering that you are starting this practice right after finishing a workout, energetically, you are already high and in your sympathetic tone. Of course, this practice also could have started with a gentler breath technique, especially if the intention isn't to do the sequence immediately after a workout. This warm-up intends to gradually bring your energy levels down by slowly adding in breath retention. After exercise, breath retention can be extra challenging due to an already increased heart rate and respiratory rate as well as EPOC. Beginning this practice with *bhastrika* can create a small carbon dioxide deficiency, making the initial breath retentions slightly more comfortable to hold. However, the rounds of *bhastrika* are kept relatively low so as not to create too much carbon dioxide deficiency in relation to the duration of the breath-holds. Ultimately, like any proper warm-up, this helps prepare you for the rest of the practice.

The warm-up begins with ten seconds of *bhastrika,* followed by an outer retention hold for fifteen seconds, directly into an inner retention hold for thirty seconds. Repeat this breath practice five times. The beginning retentions shouldn't be challenging. If the practice feels too difficult, allow a little more time for your heart rate to lower after your workout or shorten the retention.

HEAT-BUILDING

The heat-building component works into a slower breath practice with the focus on the outer retention. The breathing slows way down to about three breaths per minute, with half of the respiratory time occurring during the outer retention. The inhalations and exhalations should be only as deep as is necessary to achieve the length of the respiration. The calmer the breath, the easier it is to make the switch back to the parasympathetic nervous system. The long outer holds will quickly build up carbon dioxide levels and facilitate the expansion of the blood vessels, the increase of blood flow, and higher oxygen cellular perfusion. The parasympathetic nervous system will start to slow the heart rate and move the body into a recovery state. This breath practice consists of a five-second inhalation, a five-second exhalation, and a ten-second outer retention. Repeat this breath about fifteen times, or for approximately five minutes.

VITALIZING

The vitalizing component is a slow build from the heat-building component. The primary intention is to increase parasympathetic tone and build up carbon dioxide, which is relatively easy to do with the breath and can be carried out in several ways. The main approaches are through slowing the respiratory rate and lengthening the breath retentions. With this practice, you don't want to focus too much on long holds. It's more beneficial to use shorter retentions so that you can maintain a sustained slow breathing practice without feeling the urge to "catch your breath." It is common to over-breathe during physical exercise. You want to reestablish a slower breathing pattern as you move into recovery. This breath practice alternates between inner and outer retentions. You get more benefit from outer retention; however, outer retention can be difficult to maintain. Switching between inner and outer retentions allows for intermittent "rest" without compromising the breathing rate or carbon dioxide retention. Maintain the five-second inhalation and exhalation duration and alternate between one breath with a twenty-second inner retention and the next breath with a fifteen-second outer retention. This brings the rate down to about two breaths per minute. Maintain this breath pattern for about ten cycles, or approximately five minutes.

COOL-DOWN

The cool-down uses a descending *sama vritti* breath with *bhramari* during the exhalation. Energetically, the goal is to finish the practice in a calm and balanced state. *Sama vritti* is an excellent exercise for regulating the autonomic nervous system. The practice begins with a fifteen-second inhalation followed by a fifteen-second exhalation with the humming *bhramari* breath to increase nitric oxide levels. With each breath, decrease the ratio by 1:1 until you reach a breath ratio of 5:5. As the breath duration becomes shorter, also work to soften the intensity and depth of each respiration so that you finish in a rested and rejuvenated state.

AN OPPORTUNITY FOR BETTERMENT

Life presents us with many obstacles to navigate through or overcome. Each time we meet resistance or struggle, life offers us a new opportunity for growth. But facing challenges doesn't mean we will overcome them, and overcoming them doesn't promise we will grow from them. Stress and difficulty are required for growth; however, overcoming challenges isn't necessary for us to evolve through the experience. We often seek challenges if we are not finding them in our daily lives. Even though we all love things that give us comfort and pleasure, those things rarely give us the opportunity for betterment. Have you ever returned from a vacation of sipping drinks by the pool, lounging all day without a care in the world, and thought, "Wow, I've really grown as a person"? Probably not. But we've all faced loss, heartache, disappointment, pain, and grief, and depending on how we handled those situations, they allowed us to grow or break. Every relationship I've had that ended in heartache has made me a better person. While this might not be the best example, almost all of us have gone through experiences such as these and changed for the better. I faced death and lost friends while fighting in Iraq. That experience changed me, but most people can't relate to this beyond what we see depicted in movies. Some of my friends who fought beside me didn't grow but rather continue to suffer from that experience.

Sometimes a situation is beyond our capabilities to handle, and it creates suffering we cannot overcome, but it is not the severity of the event that decides, but how we face it. Some of the most inspiring people who have ever walked this planet were challenged in ways that would break most of us, yet they conquered, and through the tragedies they became the people we venerate. It is not the severity of the problems we face in life—to live is to know pain and loss—but how we act in situations of chaos and calamity that genuinely defines who we are. Even if those situations are mundane struggles of trying to pay bills when we don't have the money, showing up to a job we dislike, or dealing with health problems or injuries, we have a choice regarding how we see the situation and which path we take.

It's usually not a massive event like war, the death of a loved one, a divorce, or a pandemic that breaks us. We know we can survive these challenges. It's the small ongoing battles that have no end in sight that bring us to our knees and cripple our spirit. I had a tough childhood, or at least I perceived it as hard. For children, how good or bad the situation ultimately was has less significance than how they emotionally remember that situation. The same is true for adults. But as a child, I hated my life. I suffered from depression and panic attacks. I never told anyone about my struggles, and in turn, I never received help. The only thing that kept me going was that I knew that whatever my situation was, it would eventually change. As I got older and gained more control over my life, I realized I could change any situation that caused me grief and suffering. There are times when we need to face challenges and endure the struggles of daily life because they are a part of life, but we don't need to suffer; instead, we can grow because of those struggles. Every obstacle we face is a fork in the road requiring us to decide how to proceed. While the right choice might not always be clear, we can almost always turn around and choose a different outcome.

We are fortunate to have tools to help us navigate through pain, challenge, and uncertainty. The unknown will always create the biggest fear. But until we breathe our last breath and step into the great unknown, the breath remains the one certainty to guide us safely along our course.

Even before I knew anything about the breath and its vast capabilities, I knew that when life brought me to the edge, my breath would bring me back. These breath sequences are tools for living. Sometimes they can act as a map to bring us back on course, and sometimes they can act as a vehicle to carry us beyond our limits. The sequences I have shared with you can be used as suggested, transformed for other intentions, or serve as scaffolds for you to create your own breath sequences to help you navigate your life.

The concepts, physiology, philosophies, and practices in this book are resources that we can use to create positive change. Breathing is not a practice; it is a requirement for life. Learning to breathe right is preventive medicine for the mind and body. And just like every challenge gives us the opportunity for betterment, so does every breath.

NOTES

[1]Shahriar Sakhaei, Hassan E. Sadagheyani, Soryya Zinalpoor, Abdolah K. Markani, and Hossein Motaarefi, "The impact of pursed-lips breathing maneuver on cardiac, respiratory, and oxygenation parameters in COPD patients," *Open Access Macedonian Journal of Medical Sciences* 6, no. 10 (2018): 1851–6, doi:10.3889/oamjms.2018.407.

[2]Julio Fernandez-Mendoza, Fan He, Alexandros N. Vgontzas, Duanping Liao, and Edward O. Bixler, "Interplay of objective sleep duration and cardiovascular and cerebrovascular diseases on cause-specific mortality," *Journal of the American Heart Association* 8, no. 20 (2019): e013043, doi: 10.1161/JAHA.119.013043.

[3]Jane Digby, "Trouble sleeping? Learn how long caffeine stays in your system," PrepScholar blog, Oct. 16, 2017, https://blog.prepscholar.com/how-long-does-caffeine-stay-in-your-system.

[4]Ruben Meerman and Andrew J. Brown, "When somebody loses weight, where does the fat go?" *British Medical Journal* 349 (2014): g7257, doi: 10.1136/bmj.g7257.

[5]"Catabolism," in Boundless Microbiology, Lumen Learning, https://courses.lumenlearning.com/boundless-microbiology/chapter/catabolism/.

[6]J. Laforgia, R. T. Withers, N. J. Shipp, and C. J. Gore, "Comparison of energy expenditure elevations after submaximal and supramaximal running," *Journal of Applied Physiology* 82, no. 2 (1997): 661–6, doi: 10.1152/jappl.1997.82.2.661.

[7]Elisabet Borsheim and Roald Bahr, "Effect of exercise intensity, duration and mode on post-exercise oxygen consumption," *Sports Medicine* 33, no. 14 (2003): 1037–60, doi: 10.2165/00007256-200333140-00002.

[8]Lidiane I. Filippin, Andrea J. Moreira, Norma P. Marroni, and Ricardo M. Xavier, "Nitric oxide and repair of skeletal muscle injury," *Nitric Oxide* 21, no. 3–4 (2009): 157–63, doi: 10.1016/j.niox.2009.08.002; J. E. Anderson, "A role for nitric oxide in muscle repair: nitric oxide-mediated activation of muscle satellite cells," *Molecular Biology of the Cell* 11, no. 5 (2000): 1859–74, doi:10.1091/mbc.11.5.1859.

EPILOGUE:
LEARNING TO BREATHE

"I feel like I can finally breathe" and "I feel like I'm suffocating!" are common sayings to express how we feel. The breath goes beyond biological needs and is ingrained in our emotional experience. Every experience we have is centered around the way we feel about what we are experiencing. Our memories are formed from how we feel about a situation rather than the situation itself. It's this emotional imprint that shapes how we experience reality.

However, reality is an interesting concept. It refers to the state of something being real, regardless of our experience. Reality implies that what we know to be true exists independently of our ideas; it separates what *is* real from what might only appear real. It is the antithesis of fantasy. No one has ever experienced reality. We think we have, but all we know is a subjective individual viewpoint of what we conceptualize to be true.

Imagine you were born wearing a pair of glasses with blue lenses, but you didn't know you had these tinted glasses on, and even if you did, you could never take them off. Everything you saw was blue, so you thought everything was blue. You assumed that everyone else saw the world in the same hue as you, but they all had their own colored glasses on and saw the world through their special lenses. With everyone seeing the world differently and no one being able to view it without these colored glasses on, unaware of the tint of their own lenses, how would we know the actual color of the sky, the trees, or anything else? Yet we think we know reality because of what we see and experience. What we see is only a subjective reality, which isn't real, because as soon as we're gone, that reality is also gone. Actual reality exists outside of our experiences and continues with or without us.

Our perceptions are relative to our interpretations of our life experiences. We form beliefs by experiencing the spectrum of existence. We conclude what something is by determining what it is not. The essence of definition is to create separation. Black is not white, hot is not cold, light is not dark, good is not bad, and *I am not you.* I am not implying that reality is binary or that I am not you. I'm stating that what we think we know to be true is based on the concept of separation, and because we view ourselves as separate, our ability to experience anything different is limited.

Two things form our perception of reality: our preferences and our perspective. Our preferences are merely the things we desire or dislike. Our perspective is our unique view of the world. We are all having personal experiences, and because of that, everything we know or identify with comes from our unique encounters, our observations, and the knowledge or wisdom we have gained. We can never understand how someone else is experiencing life because we will never share their perception of that experience. Even if you and I go through the same event, we will experience it differently.

If you and I eat the same meal, for example, I will never know what you are tasting, even though I might *think* I know what you should like. Have you ever been out to eat with someone who makes you taste something because they think you should like it, even though they already know you don't? We assume we know what others should do, think, or believe because we think we know what is best. But our perspective inhibits us from truly understanding what others like, want, or need. For example, a person who is born blind will never experience what it's like to be in the dark. Without the reference of light, darkness doesn't exist. Yet we might pity someone who is blind because we assume that being able to see is better. Our perception makes us think we know best based on our experiences and understanding, and it makes it easy to want to push our opinions, our beliefs, and often our fears on others.

Even the words we use often come from the assumption that we define them the same way. When I started becoming well known as a yoga teacher, I was often criticized for what I was doing. My physical yoga practice is dynamic, with many arm balances, handstands, and challenging transitions that most people can't do. When I post photos or videos of my practice on social media, people tell me that what I am doing is not yoga; it's circus or gymnastics.

Because I have devoted so much time and effort to my practice, I felt like I knew what yoga was. I found these criticisms insulting and felt like I needed to defend myself and defend yoga. I would quote famous yoga teachers like Pattabhi Jois, who said, "Yoga is an internal practice. The rest is just circus." I needed to justify what I knew to be right. I had been studying and practicing yoga for years, learned from teachers who had famous lineages, and read dozens of books on the subject. What gave these people the right to tell me that what I was doing wasn't yoga? The real questions should have been, Why did I care? What did I have to prove? And, were my critics wrong?

They weren't wrong, and neither was I. I have my beliefs based on my experiences, which define my understanding of reality...and so does everyone else. When I started yoga, it was a physical practice and not much more for me. That doesn't mean that it wasn't yoga or that moving into the depths of yogic philosophy and spirituality makes it more yoga. It would be the same if I thought that only I understood the true meaning of love, and unless people saw it the way I did, they didn't really know what love was.

If we believe something to be true, and truly believe it, then there is no reason to defend it. What we are defending is our ego because what we believe in becomes the thing we attach our identity to. Our beliefs form our ego, and our experiences define our beliefs. So, when someone disagrees with how we define what we believe in, it feels personal. But their definition will always be different because it is shaped by their experiences, which are obviously unique to them.

Everyone has the right to define things as they like. When we talk about different things but use the same words, conversations can be confusing. This happens all the time, and it often creates conflict when it really is a lack of understanding. Instead of pushing our ideas, beliefs, and definitions on one another, we need to recognize that the way we understand reality is not *the* reality, only *our* reality. When we can broaden our view and see that we have a very narrow perspective of what we think we know, we can give others space to have their views without thinking we know what is best or most important.

What we value as important shapes our choices, actions, and beliefs. The truth is, nothing is important—not life, the environment, or the existence of the universe—until we decide it's important. What we value is personal. Unfortunately, we don't all share the same values, but on the other side of that coin, it's good that we don't. Of course, we all want the world to share the same values as us, but we wouldn't want to share the values of someone who doesn't have a regard for human life or the world we inhabit. Our values, morals, desires, and aversions come from the preferences that we have formed throughout our lives—some through choices of our own, but many adopted from our families, friends, and culture. We are taught what we should like and what we should want. It's crazy to imagine that a lot of our dreams and desires, especially the ones formed in childhood, were given to us. Of course, some preferences are our own, but how many have we acquired from the people who influenced us early on? Maybe a dislike for a certain food might be personal, but different cultures have unique preferences when it comes to food. Things like hate, racism, and bigotry are preferences that are learned. Nelson Mandela said, "No one is born hating another person because of the color of his skin, or his background, or his religion. People must learn to hate...." We can end racism in one generation if we teach our children to love each other and not see one another as being less just because we are different. We all look different; it's the preferences we place on that difference that make it good or bad.

Our preferences dictate which things bring us joy or create our unhappiness. The more preferences we have, the more our perspective of life rigidifies under our wants, making the beauty of an unpredictable existence impossible to enjoy. How we choose to see the world is different from how we choose to live in it. And although we are all having individual experiences, we are living in the same world and breathing the same air. Different doesn't mean separate. We feel separate because our experiences give us unique perspectives. It is only because our perspectives are limited that we are unable to see the bigger picture. We are all climbing a mountain, each of us on our own path, heading toward the summit. If we walk up the mountain looking only at our feet, we might think our path is the only path. If we look up and see one another, however, we recognize that there are as many ways up as there are people climbing. *Only when we move past our singular perspective can we realize that there aren't many paths leading to one peak, but instead only one mountain, and all of us are sharing the same journey, just seeing in different ways.* We are all different, but we are all connected, not only in life but also in our journey within it.

Learning to breathe is like learning to live. The smallest details hold the most significance. A single step in an epic adventure carries with it all the subtleties of experience that we have gained along the way. The destination is just one more step in the perpetual cycle of inhalations and exhalations. Each breath contains all the potential of life, and we can't hold either one forever. Maybe by learning to breathe, we can discover living. We're guaranteed only two breaths in this life: our first and our last. We can waste every breath merely existing, or we can use every breath to create meaning and experience the true miracle of living.

INDEX

mechanoreceptors, 49–50

men, 27–29

mental aspect, of *gunas,* 74

middle lobe, 27

mitochondria, in cellular respiration, 16

monthly cycle, of *gunas,* 74

mouth breathing, 22–23

mudras. See also specific mudras
    in breath sequence wave, 174–175, 176
    defined, 94
    jnana, 134
    nadi shodhana pranayama (alternate nostril breathing) and, 133
    shanmukhi, 145–146
    Vishnu, 134

mula bandha (root lock), 100–101

muscles, of respiration, 30–32

N

nadi shodhana pranayama (alternate nostril breathing)
    about, 65–66, 132–136
    combined with *bhramari pranayama* (humming bee breath), 167–168
    in Concentration and Memory breath sequence, 208, 211
    effects of, 154–155, 160, 164
    in Equanimity breath sequence, 181, 182
    gunas, vayus and, 162
    in Libido and Sexual Arousal breath sequence, 228, 229
    nadis and, 161
    in Sleep breath sequence, 203, 204

nadis (channels of energy), 64–68, 84

nasal breathing, 23–26

nasal cavity, 24, 25

nasal cycle, 23

nasopharynx, 24

neck, breathing and, 42

neurotransmitter, nitric oxide as a, 25

nitric oxide
    bhramari pranayama (humming bee breath) and, 144
    significance of, 24–26

nostrils, 24

O

ocean breath. *See ujjayi pranayama* (victorious breath)

oropharynx, 24

outer retention. *See bahya kumbhaka* (outer retention)

over-breathing (hyperventilation). *See also specific exercises*
    about, 18–23
    carbon dioxide and, 111
    compared with over-eating, 39
    effects of, 35
    high-altitude training and, 36–37
    in yoga, 37–39

oxygen
    in carbonic-bicarbonate buffer system, 18–19
    in cellular respiration, 16

oxygen saturation, 20

P

paranasal sinuses, 25, 145

parasympathetic nervous system, 50–53, 59, 86

passive channel. *See ida nadi* (left-side energy)

pectoralis muscle, 31

pelvis
    breathing and, 42
    mula bandha (root lock) for, 100–101

perception of reality, 241

peripheral capillary oxygen saturation (SpO_2), 20–22

peripheral nervous system, 48–50

perspective, perception of reality and, 241

pH levels
    carbonic-bicarbonate buffer system and, 18

R

rajas guna ("to do")
    about, 72
    agnisar pranayama (fire essence breath) and, 150
    attributes of, 71
    bhastrika pranayama (bellows breath) and, 126
    in breath sequence wave, 172, 173, 175
    characteristics of, 85
    in Energy Boost breath sequence, 188, 190, 192
    in *gunas* cycle, 75–76
    in Libido and Sexual Arousal breath sequence, 228, 229
    nadi shodhana pranayama (alternate nostril breathing) and, 134
    in systems of balance, 86
    ujjayi pranayama (victorious breath) and, 110–111
reality, perception of, 241
rechaka (exhalation)
    actions of, 42
    in breath cycle, 95–96
    in systems of balance, 86
    ujjayi pranayama (victorious breath) and, 109
rectus abdominis, 31
residual volume, 29, 30
"rest and digest," 50–53
retention. *See kumbhaka* (retention)
right-side energy. *See pingala nadi* (right-side energy)
root *chakra (muladhara chakra),* 69
Rosenberg, Stanley, 193

S

safe, feeling, 59–60
sama vritti pranayama (equal ratio breathing)
    about, 114–117
    effects of, 154–155, 160, 164
    in Equanimity breath sequence, 181, 183

    gunas, vayus and, 162
    in Libido and Sexual Arousal breath sequence, 228
    in Metabolism and Weight Loss breath sequence, 222, 224
    nadis and, 161
    in Post-Workout Recovery breath sequence, 234, 236
    in Sleep breath sequence, 203
    in Stress and Anxiety Relief breath sequence, 196
samana vayu
    about, 78, 82–83, 85
    pranayama practices for, 162
    in systems of balance, 86
sattva guna ("to be")
    about, 71–72, 161
    attributes of, 71
    in breath sequence wave, 172, 173–174, 175
    characteristics of, 85
    in Concentration and Memory breath sequence, 208, 210, 211
    in Equanimity breath sequence, 180
    in *gunas* cycle, 75–76
    nadi shodhana pranayama (alternate nostril breathing) and, 134
    sama vritti pranayama (equal ratio breathing) and, 115, 116
    in systems of balance, 86
scalene muscle, 31
"second wind," 37
secondary bronchus, 27
self, 91
sensory function, 49–50, 66–67
serotonin, 67
serratus anterior, 31
Severinsen, Stig, 28
sex drive, 26
sexual function, 26
shanmukhi mudra (six-gate seal), *bhramari pranayama* (humming bee breath) and, 145–146

Shiva Samhita, 67

shoulders, breathing and, 42, 43–44

signal function, of somatic nervous system, 50

simhasana pranayama, sitali and *sitkari pranayama* (cooling breath) and, 149

sitali and *sitkari pranayama* (cooling breath)
    about, 148–149
    effects of, 154–155, 160, 164
    in Energy Boost breath sequence, 190, 193
    gunas, vayus and, 162
    nadis and, 161

six-gate seal *(shanmukhi mudra),* *bhramari pranayama* (humming bee breath) and, 145–146

skull shining breath. *See kapalabhati pranayama* (skull shining breath)

Sleep breath sequence, 199–205

somatic nervous system, 49–50

sphenoid sinus, 24, 25

spine, breathing and, 42, 43

spirituality, 66, 161

sternocleidomastoid muscle, 31

stomach, posture and, 43

stress
    nitric oxide and, 26
    parasympathetic nervous system and, 51–52
    sympathetic nervous system and, 51–52

Stress and Anxiety Relief breath sequence, 194–199

stress response, 59–60

superior lobe, 27

sushumna nadi
    about, 69–70, 84, 161
    effects of, 68
    in Equanimity breath sequence, 180
    pranayama practices for, 161
    in systems of balance, 86

sympathetic nervous system, 50–53, 60, 84, 86

system of relationships. *See prana vayus* (system of relationships)

systems of balance
    about, 47–48, 86
    autonomic nervous system, 55–64
    combining, 83–86
    gunas (expressions of energy), 70–76
    nadis (channels of energy), 65–70
    polyvagal theory, 55–64
    prana vayus (system of relationships), 77–83
    pranayama practices, 154–155

T

tamas guna ("to have")
    about, 73
    attributes of, 71
    in breath sequence wave, 175
    characteristics of, 85
    in *gunas* cycle, 75–76
    nadi shodhana pranayama (alternate nostril breathing) and, 134
    in Sleep breath sequence, 204, 205
    in Stress and Anxiety Relief breath sequence, 198
    in systems of balance, 86
    vishama vritti pranayama (unequal ratio breathing) and, 120

tertiary bronchus, 27

thermal energy, 67

thermodynamics, law of, 220

third eye *chakra (ajna chakra),* 69

thoracic cavity, 28, 30

three-part breathing. *See dirgha svasam pranayama* (three-part breathing)

throat *chakra (vishuddha), jalandhara bandha* (throat lock) and, 102

throat lock. *See jalandhara bandha* (throat lock)

tidal volume, 28–29, 30–31, 98

tongue, 24

trachea, 24, 27

training, at high elevation, 36

transverse abdominis, 31
triangle pose, *ujjayi* breath and, 37

U

udana vayu
  about, 78, 80–81, 85
  nadi shodhana pranayama (alternate nostril breathing) and, 132
  pranayama practices for, 162
  in systems of balance, 86
  uddiyana bandha (abdominal lock) and, 101–102
uddiyana bandha (abdominal lock)
  about, 100, 101–102
  agnisar pranayama (fire essence breath) and, 150
  in Concentration and Memory breath sequence, 209, 211
  kapalabhati pranayama (skull shining breath) and, 122
  in Metabolism and Weight Loss breath sequence, 223
ujjayi pranayama (victorious breath)
  about, 37–38, 108–113, 157
  bhramari pranayama (humming bee breath) and, 145
  effects of, 154–155, 160, 164
  in Energy Boost breath sequence, 190, 192
  in Libido and Sexual Arousal breath sequence, 228, 229, 230
  nadi shodhana pranayama (alternate nostril breathing) and, 135
  nadis and, 161
  pranayama practices for, 162
  sama vritti pranayama (equal ratio breathing) and, 114, 116
under-breathing (hypoventilation). *See also specific exercises*
  benefits of, 34–35
  effects of, 35
  high-altitude training and, 36–37
unequal ratio breathing. *See vishama vritti pranayama* (unequal ratio breathing)

the unspoken mantra (*ajapa* mantra), *ujjayi pranayama* (victorious breath) and, 109
upper respiratory system, 23–24

V

vagus nerve, 52, 53–54
Valsalva maneuver, 111, 112
vasodilator, nitric oxide as a, 25–26
vayus
  in breath sequence wave, 174–175
  pranayama practices for, 162
ventral vagal complex, 54, 60, 84, 86
vestibular fold, 24
victorious breath. *See ujjayi pranayama* (victorious breath)
viloma pranayama (interrupted breathing)
  about, 137–144
  effects of, 154–155, 160, 164
  in Energy Boost breath sequence, 190, 192
  in Equanimity breath sequence, 181, 183
  for health-related goals, 163
  nadis and, 161
  for physical goals, 163
  pranayama practices for, 162
vishama vritti pranayama (unequal ratio breathing)
  about, 118–121
  in Concentration and Memory breath sequence, 208
  effects of, 154–155, 160, 164
  in Libido and Sexual Arousal breath sequence, 228, 229, 230
  in Metabolism and Weight Loss breath sequence, 222, 224
  nadis and, 161
  in Post-Workout Recovery breath sequence, 234
  pranayama practices for, 162
  in Sleep breath sequence, 203
  in Stress and Anxiety Relief breath sequence, 198

ABOUT THE AUTHOR

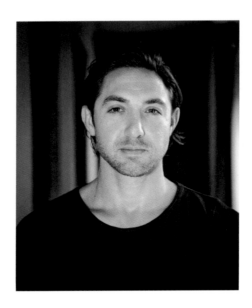

Dylan Werner is a renowned international yoga instructor, lecturer, and educator in health, well-being, and mindfulness. His extensive knowledge of anatomy and physiology and deep understanding of Eastern philosophy lend a unique perspective to his teachings. A former United States Marine and Iraq War veteran turned city firefighter/paramedic, Dylan left his career to pursue a life of mindfulness, dedicating himself to helping others in their journey toward a more peaceful, harmonious life.